OVERCOMING PORN ADDICTION FOR YOUNG ADULTS

A Guide to Breaking Free and Understanding Yourself

William L. Garris

TABLE OF CONTENTS

INTRODUCTION

In a world inundated with information and digital distractions, young adults are increasingly confronted with challenges that previous generations never had to face. Among these challenges, one stands out for its profound impact on mental, emotional, and even physical well-being: porn addiction. This is a topic often shrouded in secrecy, shame, and misunderstanding, yet it affects millions of young adults globally. You are not alone.

Welcome to "Overcoming Porn Addiction for Young Adults: A Guide to Breaking Free and Understanding Yourself." This book is your companion on a journey towards liberation, self-discovery, and a healthier relationship with your mind and body. I'm here to guide you, not as an expert who has all the answers, but as someone who understands the struggle and the path to overcoming it.

Why This Book?
You might be wondering why you should invest your time in reading this book. After all, there are countless resources available online about addiction and self-help. But let me tell you a little secret: this book is different.

It's not just another manual filled with dry facts and statistics. This book is a heartfelt guide written specifically for you a young adult navigating the complexities of modern life, grappling with desires, temptations, and the quest for self-understanding.

I've crafted this book to resonate with your unique experiences and emotions. It's designed to address the specific challenges you face as a young adult dealing with porn addiction. Here, you will find not only practical steps to overcome addiction but also insights into understanding yourself better, reclaiming your power, and transforming your life.

A Personal Journey
Let's face it: talking about porn addiction isn't easy. It's a topic that many avoid due to embarrassment or fear of judgment. But acknowledging the problem is the first step towards healing. I remember feeling isolated, ashamed, and powerless when I first confronted my addiction. It was like being trapped in a vicious cycle that seemed impossible to break.

But then, something changed. I began to understand that addiction isn't just about willpower; it's about understanding the underlying issues that drive the behavior. It's about recognizing the patterns and triggers that keep you hooked and learning how to navigate them.

Most importantly, it's about realizing that you have the strength within you to overcome this.

Breaking Free
Breaking free from porn addiction is not an overnight miracle. It's a journey that requires patience, commitment, and, most importantly, self-compassion. This book is structured to help you take that journey step by step. We'll start by understanding what porn addiction is and how it affects your brain and body. We'll explore the psychological and emotional factors that contribute to addiction, and you'll learn practical strategies to break free.

You'll find exercises and activities designed to help you reflect on your experiences, identify your triggers, and develop healthier coping mechanisms. You'll also discover stories of others who have successfully overcome their addictions, providing inspiration and a sense of solidarity.

Understanding Yourself
Understanding yourself is a crucial part of overcoming addiction. Why do we turn to porn? What are we seeking when we do? Often, addiction is a way to escape from deeper issues such as stress, loneliness, anxiety, or low self-esteem. This book will guide you in exploring these

underlying issues and help you build a stronger, more resilient sense of self.

We'll delve into mindfulness practices, emotional intelligence, and self-care techniques that can help you reconnect with your inner self. By understanding your thoughts, feelings, and behaviors, you'll be better equipped to make conscious choices that align with your true values and aspirations.

The Power of Connection

One of the most powerful tools in overcoming addiction is connection. Addiction thrives in isolation, and breaking free requires reaching out and building supportive relationships. Throughout this book, you'll find encouragement to connect with others – whether it's through support groups, therapy, or trusted friends and family.

You'll learn how to communicate your struggles and seek help without fear of judgment. By sharing your journey, you'll not only find strength but also help others who are facing similar challenges.

Your Journey Starts Here

As you embark on this journey, remember that you are not defined by your addiction. You are a complex, multifaceted individual with immense potential. This book is here to remind you of that potential and to support you in unlocking it.

Every chapter, every exercise, and every story in this book is designed with one goal in mind: to help you break free from porn addiction and understand yourself better. It's a journey that will challenge you, but it's also one that will transform you.

So, take a deep breath, open your mind, and dive in. Your journey to breaking free and understanding yourself starts here. Let's walk this path together, one step at a time, towards a brighter, healthier future.

Chapter 1

Understanding the Rising Concern of Porn Addiction in Young Adult

Porn addiction in young adults is a growing concern that has emerged in the digital age due to the widespread availability of explicit content on the internet. With just a few clicks or taps, young people can access a vast array of sexually explicit material through websites, social media platforms, or mobile applications. This easy accessibility and anonymity make it challenging for individuals to resist the temptation, leading to the development of addictive behaviors.

Addiction to porn can have significant implications on various aspects of a young adult's life:

Mental Health: Excessive consumption of porn can lead to feelings of guilt, shame, and anxiety. It can alter brain chemistry and dopamine levels, reinforcing the desire for more explicit content, and potentially leading to an unhealthy dependence on it to cope with stress or emotions.Dopamine and Reward System: Viewing explicit content can trigger the brain's reward system, leading to the release of dopamine - a neurotransmitter associated with pleasure and reinforcement. Over time, the brain may become desensitized to the same level of stimulation, leading to an increased desire for more explicit or novel material to achieve the same dopamine response. This cycle can foster addictive behaviors, as individuals seek out more and more pornographic content.

Escapism and Coping Mechanism: Porn addiction can develop as a form of escapism from stress, anxiety, or emotional pain. Young adults may turn to pornography as a way to numb negative emotions temporarily. However, this coping mechanism can be harmful in the long run, as it prevents them from addressing the root causes of their distress and finding healthier ways to cope.

Emotional Consequences: Regular exposure to explicit content can lead to feelings of guilt, shame, and self-esteem issues, especially if individuals perceive their behavior as morally wrong or in conflict with their values. These negative emotions can further perpetuate the addictive cycle, as individuals may use porn to alleviate these negative feelings.

Impact on Relationships: Porn addiction can interfere with real-life relationships. Young adults who are addicted to porn may struggle to establish emotional connections with their partners, as they may prioritize their virtual experiences over genuine intimacy. This can lead to feelings of alienation, mistrust, and dissatisfaction in their relationships.

Mental Health Disorders: Porn addiction may exacerbate or contribute to the development of mental health disorders, such as depression and anxiety. The constant pursuit of explicit content can become a compulsive behavior that interferes with daily life and responsibilities.

Distorted Views of Sexuality: Frequent exposure to unrealistic portrayals of sex in pornography can lead to distorted views of sexuality and body image. Young adults may start to compare themselves or their partners to the performers in porn, which can lead to insecurities and unrealistic expectations about sex.

Addressing the mental health aspect of porn addiction involves recognizing the addictive nature of explicit content and its potential impact on emotional well-being. Encouraging young adults to seek support, whether through therapy, counseling, or support groups, can help them develop healthier coping mechanisms and strategies to overcome addiction. Promoting a non-judgmental environment for discussions about mental health and sexuality is crucial in providing the necessary guidance to navigate the challenges of excessive porn consumption.

Relationships: Porn addiction can adversely affect intimate relationships. It may lead to unrealistic expectations about sex, difficulty establishing emotional connections, and decreased sexual satisfaction with real-life partners. Trust issues and communication breakdowns may arise, further straining relationships.Unrealistic Expectations about Sex:

Regular consumption of pornography can create unrealistic expectations about sex and intimate relationships. Porn often presents idealized and scripted scenarios that don't reflect real-life experiences. This can lead to individuals expecting their partners to perform like the actors in porn, causing disappointment and dissatisfaction when reality doesn't match the fantasy.

2. Difficulty Establishing Emotional Connections:

Porn addiction can hinder the development of emotional intimacy in relationships. When one partner becomes preoccupied with explicit content, they may withdraw emotionally from their real-life partner. Emotional bonding requires open communication, empathy, and vulnerability, which can be challenging when one partner is more focused on a sexualized fantasy world.

3. Decreased Sexual Satisfaction with Real-Life Partners:

Excessive consumption of porn can lead to a reduced desire for real-life sexual intimacy. The novelty and intensity of explicit content can overshadow the intimacy shared with a partner, causing a decline in sexual satisfaction within the relationship.

4. Trust Issues:

Porn addiction may lead to trust issues in relationships. If a partner feels their significant other is secretive about their porn use or prefers it over real-life intimacy, it can erode trust and create feelings of betrayal.

5. Communication Breakdowns:

Porn addiction can hinder open communication about sexual desires and boundaries. Partners may avoid discussing their concerns or discomfort with explicit content, fearing judgment or confrontation. This lack of communication can lead to misunderstandings and distance between partners.

6. Emotional Disconnection:

Porn addiction can cause emotional disconnection between partners. Instead of seeking emotional support or companionship from their real-life partner, an individual may turn to explicit content as a coping mechanism or a substitute for genuine emotional connection.

7. Impact on Self-Esteem:

For the partner not struggling with porn addiction, knowing that their significant other is consuming explicit content excessively can negatively impact their self-esteem. They might question their attractiveness or worry about not living up to the unrealistic standards presented in porn.

To address these issues, it's essential for couples to engage in open and honest communication. Recognizing the impact of porn addiction on the relationship is the first step. Seeking professional help, such as couples therapy, can be beneficial in addressing underlying issues and developing healthier coping strategies.

Individuals struggling with porn addiction should consider seeking support through therapy, support groups, or online resources tailored to overcoming such challenges. Building awareness, understanding the potential consequences, and working together to rebuild trust and emotional intimacy can lead to healthier and more fulfilling relationships.

Physical Health: Spending long hours viewing explicit material can lead to physical issues like fatigue, disrupted sleep patterns, and reduced sexual desire with real partners.

Social Withdrawal: Addiction to porn can lead to isolation, as individuals may prefer spending time alone to engage in their habit rather than socializing or pursuing other activities.

Performance Anxiety: Regular exposure to unrealistic portrayals of sex in porn can lead to performance anxiety and insecurity in intimate situations.

Addressing this rising concern requires a multi-faceted approach:

Education and Awareness: It is crucial to educate young adults about the potential risks of porn addiction and the impact it can have on mental health, relationships, and overall well-being.

Open Dialogue: Encourage open communication about sex, relationships, and healthy boundaries with parents, mentors, or counselors, creating a safe space for discussing any concerns or questions.

Digital Literacy: Promote digital literacy and responsible internet usage among young adults, emphasizing the importance of discerning reliable sources of information and setting limits on screen time.

Therapy and Support: Professional counseling or therapy can be beneficial for those struggling with porn addiction. Support groups and online forums can also offer a sense of community and understanding.

Parental Controls and Filters: Parents and guardians can utilize parental control tools and content filters to limit access to explicit content, especially for younger users.

Healthy Coping Mechanisms: Encourage the development of healthy coping mechanisms for stress and emotions, such as engaging in physical activities, hobbies, or spending quality time with loved ones.

By addressing the rising concern of porn addiction in young adults through education, communication, and support, we can work towards creating a healthier and more balanced digital environment for the next generation.

The Impact of Pornography on Brain Health and Mental Well-being

The impact of pornography on brain health and mental well-being is a complex and evolving area of research. While some studies suggest potential negative effects, the research is not definitive and requires further investigation. Here are some key points to consider:

1. Dopamine and Reward System:

Pornography can trigger the brain's reward system, leading to the release of dopamine, a neurotransmitter associated with pleasure and reinforcement. Frequent exposure to explicit content can cause desensitization, leading individuals to seek more explicit or extreme material to achieve the same level of pleasure, similar to how drug addiction works.Dopamine is a neurotransmitter that plays a key role in the brain's reward system. It is associated with feelings of pleasure, motivation, and reinforcement. When we experience something pleasurable or rewarding, such as eating delicious food or engaging in enjoyable activities, dopamine is released in the brain, creating a sense of satisfaction and encouraging us to seek out similar experiences in the future.

2. Dopamine Release and Pornography:

Watching pornography can also trigger the release of dopamine in the brain. The explicit and sexually stimulating content can activate the reward circuitry, leading to feelings of pleasure and arousal. This dopamine release is a natural and evolutionary mechanism that reinforces behaviors necessary for survival and reproduction.

3. Desensitization and Tolerance:

With repeated exposure to pornography, some individuals may experience desensitization, where the brain becomes less responsive to the same level of dopamine release. As a result, they may seek more explicit or extreme content to achieve the same level of pleasure they initially experienced. This process is similar to the development of tolerance seen in drug addiction.

4. Potential for Addiction-like Behaviors:

The combination of frequent dopamine surges and the ease of access to a vast array of explicit content on the internet can lead to compulsive behavior in some individuals. This is where the line between casual consumption and addiction can blur.

5. Pornography Addiction and Brain Changes:

Studies using brain imaging techniques have shown that individuals with pornography addiction may exhibit alterations in brain activity and connectivity, particularly in regions associated with motivation, decision-making, and impulse control. These changes may be similar to those observed in other forms of behavioral addiction and substance use disorders.

6. Individual Differences:

It's essential to recognize that not everyone who watches pornography will experience addiction or significant changes in brain activity. Individual susceptibility to addiction can vary based on factors such as genetics, environmental influences, and personal coping mechanisms.

7. Challenging Research Area:

Studying the impact of pornography on the brain is complex due to ethical considerations and methodological challenges. Longitudinal studies are challenging to conduct, and it's difficult to establish causality definitively.

It's important to note that not all individuals who view pornography will develop addiction or experience negative consequences. For many people, porn consumption is a normal part of their sexual experiences and does not lead to adverse effects on their well-being.

The key takeaway is that while pornography can trigger dopamine release and stimulate the brain's reward system, the extent and impact of this stimulation depend on individual responses, consumption patterns, and overall mental health. More research is needed to fully understand the neurological effects of pornography and its potential implications on mental well-being and addictive behaviors.

2. Changes in Brain Structure:

Some studies suggest that chronic porn use may lead to structural changes in the brain, particularly in areas related to motivation, decision-making, and impulse control. However, it's important to note that more research is needed to fully understand the extent and significance of these changes.The brain is a highly complex organ, and its structure and functioning can be influenced by various external factors, including the consumption of explicit content, such as pornography.

Some studies have indicated that chronic and excessive porn use may lead to certain changes in brain structure, particularly in areas associated with motivation, decision-making, and impulse control.

a) Dopamine and Reward Circuitry:

When individuals engage in activities that provide pleasure or reward, such as eating tasty food or experiencing intimacy, the brain releases dopamine, a neurotransmitter linked to the brain's reward system. This dopamine release reinforces the behavior, making individuals more likely to seek that pleasurable experience again.

Pornography, being a highly stimulating and novel source of sexual content, can lead to significant dopamine releases when viewed. Repeated exposure to explicit material can create a conditioned response, where the brain associates viewing porn with pleasure, encouraging individuals to seek it out more frequently.

b) Desensitization and Tolerance:

With continued and escalating porn consumption, some individuals may experience a phenomenon known as desensitization. This means that over time, the same amount or type of explicit content may not elicit the same level of pleasure as before. As a result, individuals may seek more explicit or novel content to achieve the same level of dopamine release, similar to how drug tolerance develops in substance addiction.

c) Impact on Prefrontal Cortex:

The prefrontal cortex is responsible for executive functions such as impulse control, decision-making, and goal-setting. Some studies suggest that excessive porn use could lead to reduced gray matter volume in the prefrontal cortex. This could potentially affect an individual's ability to regulate their impulses, leading to more impulsive behaviors and difficulty in making sound decisions.

d) Striatal Volume and Sensitization:

The striatum, another brain region involved in the reward system, may also undergo changes with repeated porn consumption. Some studies have found associations between larger striatal volume and higher levels of pornography consumption. This could indicate a state of sensitization, where the brain becomes more responsive to porn-related stimuli.

e) Correlation vs. Causation:

It's essential to note that while some studies have found correlations between excessive porn consumption and brain changes, causation has not been definitively established. Other factors, such as individual predispositions, co-occurring behaviors, or pre-existing brain structure, could contribute to these associations.

It is crucial to interpret these findings with caution and recognize that not all individuals who view pornography will experience significant brain changes or negative consequences. Individual responses can vary widely, and the research in this area is still relatively limited and not entirely conclusive.

As the field of neuroscience continues to advance, researchers will likely gain a more comprehensive understanding of how pornography affects the brain. In the meantime, it is essential for individuals to be aware of their own behaviors, maintain a healthy balance in their media consumption, and seek professional help if they feel their porn use is becoming problematic or affecting their well-being.
3. Mental Health Impact:

Excessive consumption of pornography has been associated with potential negative effects on mental health. Some individuals may experience feelings of guilt, shame, or anxiety related to their porn use.

Additionally, porn addiction may contribute to symptoms of depression, social anxiety, and low self-esteem in some cases.Excessive consumption of pornography has been associated with several potential negative effects on mental well-being. It's essential to remember that individual responses can vary, and not everyone who views pornography will experience these effects. However, some common mental health implications include:

a. Guilt and Shame: Viewing explicit content can trigger feelings of guilt and shame, especially if an individual holds personal or cultural beliefs that stigmatize pornography. This internal conflict can lead to emotional distress and a negative self-perception.

b. Anxiety and Obsessive Thoughts: Porn addiction can lead to anxiety and obsessive thoughts about viewing more explicit material. The compulsion to seek out pornographic content can become disruptive to daily life and lead to feelings of loss of control.

c. Negative Self-Esteem: Frequent exposure to unrealistic portrayals of sexual experiences in porn can negatively impact self-esteem. Individuals may compare themselves to the performers in explicit content and feel inadequate or insecure about their own bodies and sexual abilities.

d. Emotional Numbness: Repeated exposure to explicit content can desensitize individuals emotionally, making it challenging to connect with or empathize with others. This emotional numbing may extend to other aspects of life, affecting relationships and overall well-being.

e. Depression: Some studies have suggested a link between frequent porn consumption and symptoms of depression. The reasons for this correlation are not entirely understood and could be due to various factors, such as the impact of addiction or feelings of isolation.

f. Escapism and Coping Mechanism: Pornography can become a way for individuals to escape from stress, emotional pain, or life challenges. This reliance on explicit content as a coping mechanism may prevent individuals from addressing underlying issues effectively, leading to a cycle of dependency.

g. Distorted Perception of Sexuality: Pornography often portrays a narrow and exaggerated view of sexuality, which can shape an individual's understanding of intimate relationships. This distorted perception may lead to unrealistic expectations about sex and hinder healthy sexual development.

It's important to emphasize that not everyone who views pornography will experience these negative effects, and some individuals may have more resilience or fewer adverse consequences. The impact of pornography on mental health is highly individual and can be influenced by factors such as pre-existing mental health conditions, personal beliefs, cultural background, and the frequency and intensity of consumption.

To address potential mental health concerns related to porn consumption, individuals can consider seeking professional help from therapists or counselors specialized in sex addiction or sexual health. Developing healthy coping strategies, practicing self-awareness, and fostering open communication in relationships can also contribute to maintaining better mental well-being.
4. Relationship Distress:

As mentioned earlier, pornography addiction can negatively affect intimate relationships, leading to emotional distance, communication issues, and decreased sexual satisfaction. These relationship challenges can, in turn, impact mental well-being and overall happiness.Pornography addiction can significantly affect intimate relationships, leading to various forms of relationship distress. Here are some key aspects to consider:

Emotional Distance:

One of the primary consequences of porn addiction is emotional distance between partners. When one person becomes preoccupied with explicit content, they may emotionally withdraw from their real-life partner. Instead of seeking emotional connection and support from their significant other, they may turn to the fantasy world of pornography. This emotional disconnection can create a sense of loneliness and isolation in the relationship.

Communication Issues:

Porn addiction can hinder open and honest communication between partners about their feelings, desires, and concerns related to sex and intimacy. Individuals struggling with porn addiction may feel embarrassed or ashamed to discuss their habit with their partner, leading to a breakdown in communication. This lack of openness can prevent couples from addressing underlying issues and finding solutions together.

Decreased Sexual Satisfaction:

Excessive porn consumption can lead to a decline in sexual satisfaction within the relationship. The unrealistic portrayals of sex in pornography may create a distorted view of what sex should be like in real life. This can lead to a diminished interest in sexual intimacy with a partner, as the explicit content may become more appealing or fulfilling than real-life experiences.

Trust Issues:

Porn addiction can erode trust in a relationship. If a partner feels that their significant other is secretive about their porn use or prefers explicit content over real-life intimacy, it can lead to feelings of betrayal and insecurity. Trust is a fundamental aspect of a healthy relationship, and its erosion can have long-lasting effects.

Comparison and Insecurity:

Partners who are aware of their significant other's porn addiction may also experience feelings of comparison and insecurity. They might worry that they cannot live up to the unrealistic standards portrayed in porn, leading to a negative impact on their self-esteem and confidence.

Difficulty Establishing Emotional Intimacy:

Emotional intimacy is a vital component of a strong relationship. However, porn addiction can hinder the development of emotional connection and bonding. A person preoccupied with explicit content may find it challenging to fully engage emotionally with their partner, leading to feelings of detachment and isolation.

Addressing relationship distress caused by porn addiction requires open communication, empathy, and understanding from both partners. Seeking professional help, such as couples therapy, can be beneficial in navigating the challenges and working towards rebuilding trust and emotional intimacy.

Individuals struggling with porn addiction should also consider seeking support through therapy or support groups that specialize in addressing such issues. Openness, honesty, and a commitment to building a healthy and fulfilling relationship are essential in overcoming the impact of pornography on relationship well-being.

5. Sexual Dysfunction:

In some cases, chronic porn use has been linked to sexual dysfunction, such as erectile dysfunction or difficulty achieving orgasm. This phenomenon, known as "porn-induced erectile dysfunction," is still a subject of debate among experts, and its prevalence and causation remain unclear.Porn-induced erectile dysfunction refers to the condition where an individual, typically young men, experience difficulty achieving or maintaining an erection during sexual activity with a real-life partner, despite having no trouble during masturbation or while consuming explicit content.

Possible Mechanism:

The exact mechanisms underlying PIED are not yet fully understood and are still a subject of debate among researchers and experts. However, some theories suggest that excessive exposure to pornography may lead to:

1. Desensitization: Frequent consumption of explicit content can lead to desensitization to sexual stimuli. Over time, individuals may require increasingly intense or novel visual material to become sexually aroused.
2. Overstimulation: Pornography offers an abundance of sexual content, often presenting unrealistic and exaggerated sexual encounters. This hyper-stimulation may create a stark contrast to real-life sexual experiences, making it difficult for individuals to find real-life encounters as arousing.
3. Neuroplasticity: The brain's neuroplasticity allows it to adapt to new experiences and stimuli. Chronic porn use may lead to changes in neural pathways related to sexual arousal, potentially interfering with real-life sexual responsiveness.

Psychological Factors:

PIED can also have psychological aspects. When a person faces difficulties achieving or maintaining an erection during sexual encounters, it can lead to performance anxiety, further exacerbating the problem. The anxiety and pressure to perform can create a cycle of erectile difficulties, impacting the person's confidence and self-esteem.

Research Limitations:

It's important to note that research on PIED is still in its early stages, and the condition is not yet recognized as an official medical diagnosis. Studies exploring the link between porn consumption and erectile dysfunction have been limited in scope and often rely on self-reported data, which may introduce biases and inaccuracies.

Reversibility and Recovery:

The good news is that some evidence suggests that PIED can be reversible. By reducing or abstaining from pornography consumption, some individuals have reported improvements in their ability to achieve and maintain erections during real-life sexual encounters.

Holistic Approach:

Addressing PIED involves adopting a holistic approach. This may include reducing or eliminating porn consumption, seeking professional guidance or therapy to address psychological factors, and improving communication and intimacy with real-life partners. Developing a healthy understanding of sexuality and focusing on emotional connection rather than solely on physical performance can also be beneficial.

Individual Variability:

It's essential to recognize that not everyone who consumes explicit content will experience PIED. People's responses to porn are highly individual, and various factors, including age, frequency of consumption, and overall mental health, can play a role in determining the impact on sexual functioning.

Overall, more research is needed to better understand the complex relationship between porn consumption and erectile dysfunction. In the meantime, individuals experiencing sexual difficulties should consider seeking guidance from healthcare professionals or sex therapists who can provide personalized advice and support.
6. Addiction and Withdrawal:

Some individuals may develop compulsive behaviors and experience withdrawal-like symptoms when attempting to reduce or quit their porn consumption. This pattern of behavior is similar to substance addiction, suggesting that porn addiction could have significant consequences for mental well-being.Porn addiction, also known as compulsive sexual behavior or problematic sexual behavior, refers to a pattern of excessive and compulsive porn consumption despite negative consequences. Like other addictions, it involves a loss of control over the behavior, leading to continued engagement even when it interferes with daily life, relationships, and overall well-being.

Withdrawal-like Symptoms:

Individuals struggling with porn addiction may experience withdrawal-like symptoms when they attempt to reduce or stop their porn consumption. These symptoms can be both psychological and physiological in nature. While the exact mechanisms are not yet fully understood, some possible reasons for these symptoms include:

1. Dopamine Imbalance: Chronic exposure to pornography can create an overstimulation of the brain's reward system, leading to an increased release of dopamine during porn consumption. When individuals try to abstain, the brain experiences a temporary decrease in dopamine levels, resulting in feelings of discomfort or craving.
2. Anxiety and Irritability: Trying to abstain from porn can cause heightened anxiety and irritability, as individuals may find it challenging to cope

with the stress and emotional discomfort that arise during withdrawal.

3. Restlessness and Insomnia: Some individuals may experience difficulty falling asleep or staying asleep when trying to reduce or quit porn consumption.

4. Compulsive Behavior Relapse: During withdrawal, individuals may have intense urges or cravings to return to their porn habit as a way to alleviate the discomfort. This can result in a cycle of compulsive behavior, making it challenging to break free from the addiction.

Similarities to Substance Addiction:

The withdrawal symptoms associated with porn addiction share similarities with those seen in substance addictions. When individuals addicted to drugs or alcohol attempt to quit, they often experience withdrawal symptoms as their body and brain adjust to the absence of the substance. Similarly, those struggling with porn addiction can experience a similar withdrawal process when attempting to stop their compulsive behavior.

It's important to note that not everyone who consumes pornography will develop an addiction or experience withdrawal-like symptoms. Addiction is a complex interplay of biological, psychological, and environmental factors. Some individuals may view explicit content without experiencing any negative consequences, while others may find it challenging to control their behavior and experience distress related to their porn consumption.

As with any addiction, seeking professional help from therapists or support groups specializing in sexual addiction can be beneficial. Therapy can address underlying issues, provide coping strategies, and offer guidance on developing healthier patterns of behavior. Additionally, support from loved ones and a commitment to self awareness and personal growth can aid in the recovery process.

It's crucial to emphasize that not everyone who views pornography will experience negative effects, and individual responses can vary. Responsible and moderate porn consumption may not necessarily lead to adverse outcomes for all individuals.

Additionally, research in this area is challenging due to ethical considerations and difficulties in conducting controlled studies. Longitudinal studies examining the long-term effects of pornography on brain health and mental well-being are relatively scarce.

Overall, while some evidence suggests that excessive porn consumption may have potential negative effects on brain health and mental well-being, more research is needed to better understand the causal relationships and individual differences involved. As with any behavior, moderation, open communication, and self-awareness are essential in promoting a balanced approach to sexuality and maintaining mental well-being.

Chapter 2

Unraveling the World of Pornography

The Allure of Pornography: Psychology and Neuroscience

The allure of pornography is a complex phenomenon that involves various psychological and neurobiological factors. It captivates individuals for a combination of reasons, and understanding these factors can shed light on its appeal:

1. Instant Gratification: Pornography provides instant gratification, easily accessible through the internet and mobile devices. The brain's reward system is activated, releasing dopamine, which creates a sense of pleasure and reinforcement, leading to a desire for more.Instant gratification refers to the immediate satisfaction or

pleasure derived from a particular action or behavior. In the context of pornography, it is the quick and easy access to explicit content through the internet and mobile devices that fuels this aspect of human behavior. Several factors contribute to the allure of instant gratification in the context of pornography:

1. Accessibility and Convenience:

With the widespread availability of high-speed internet and mobile devices, accessing pornography has become incredibly easy and convenient. It takes just a few taps or clicks to find a vast array of explicit content, making it tempting for individuals seeking immediate pleasure or relief.

2. Low Effort, High Reward:

The process of accessing pornography requires minimal effort compared to other activities that might provide similar pleasure. It doesn't require social interaction or physical exertion, making it a readily available option for individuals seeking a quick reward.

3. Dopamine Release and Pleasure:

The allure of instant gratification in pornography is closely linked to the brain's reward system. When individuals engage with explicit content, their brains release dopamine, a neurotransmitter associated with pleasure and reinforcement. This release of dopamine creates a sense of enjoyment, making the behavior rewarding and reinforcing a desire for more.

4. Psychological Conditioning:

Receiving immediate pleasure from pornography can condition the brain to associate the behavior with positive outcomes. Over time, this psychological conditioning strengthens the allure of seeking instant gratification through pornography.

5. Escapism and Stress Relief:

The instant gratification provided by pornography can act as a form of escapism, offering a quick distraction from stress, boredom, or negative emotions. This escape can be alluring, as individuals may seek relief from life's challenges or emotional discomfort.

While seeking instant gratification through pornography may provide momentary pleasure, it's important to consider its potential negative effects on mental health, relationships, and overall well-being. Excessive and compulsive consumption of explicit content can lead to addiction, desensitization, relationship issues, and other adverse consequences.

Promoting awareness of the allure of instant gratification and its potential impact is crucial in fostering responsible internet usage and promoting healthier coping mechanisms. Encouraging a balanced approach to sexuality, maintaining open communication, and seeking support when necessary can aid in mitigating the potential negative effects of seeking instant gratification through pornography.

2. Novelty and Variety: The vast array of explicit content available online offers novelty and variety, triggering curiosity and exploration. This novelty-seeking behavior is a fundamental aspect of human psychology.Novelty and variety play significant roles in the allure of pornography due to their influence on human psychology. These factors tap into the fundamental human tendency to seek out new experiences and stimuli. Here's a more detailed explanation:

1. Curiosity and Exploration:

Humans are naturally curious beings. We seek out new and unfamiliar experiences to stimulate our minds and satisfy our curiosity. The vast array of explicit content available online offers an almost endless variety of scenarios, themes, and actors, catering to diverse interests and preferences. This variety piques curiosity and encourages exploration as individuals may be drawn to explore different types of content.

2. Dopaminergic Response to Novelty:

The brain's reward system responds to novelty with increased dopamine release. Dopamine is a neurotransmitter associated with pleasure and motivation. When individuals encounter something new or exciting, such as novel explicit content, it triggers a surge of dopamine, which reinforces the desire to seek out more of these experiences. This response fuels a cycle of seeking novel content to experience the pleasure associated with dopamine release.

3. Satiation and Sensitization:

Novelty-seeking behavior can also influence how individuals respond to explicit content over time. Initially, new experiences can be highly rewarding, leading to intense arousal and interest. However, with repeated exposure to the same content, the brain can become desensitized to its effects. This process is called "sensitization," where individuals may need more explicit or novel material to achieve the same level of arousal they experienced initially. This cycle of seeking novel experiences to maintain arousal can contribute to compulsive behavior and the allure of pornography.

4. The Internet's Role in Amplifying Novelty:

The internet has revolutionized access to explicit content. Unlike traditional media, the internet offers an immense and constantly updating pool of material, making it easier for individuals to find new and diverse content. This constant stream of novelty can keep individuals engaged and fuel their curiosity.

5. Reinforcement Learning:

The allure of novelty and variety in pornography is further reinforced through a process called reinforcement learning. When individuals encounter new content that aligns with their preferences or desires, it reinforces their behavior of seeking out explicit material. This process strengthens the association between novelty-seeking and explicit content consumption, contributing to the allure and potential addiction.

It's important to recognize that while novelty and variety are natural aspects of human psychology, excessive consumption of explicit content can lead to negative consequences, such as addiction, relationship issues, and potential impacts on mental health. Practicing moderation, being mindful of the influence of novelty-seeking behavior, and seeking help if one feels their consumption is becoming problematic can help maintain a healthier relationship with explicit content and overall well-being.

3. Escapism and Stress Relief: Pornography can serve as a form of escapism, providing an outlet to temporarily escape from stress, boredom, or negative emotions. It offers a brief respite from real-life challenges.Escapism and stress relief are two significant psychological factors that contribute to the allure of pornography for some individuals. Here's a more detailed explanation of how pornography can serve as a means of escape and stress relief:

1. Escape from Real-Life Challenges:

Life can be filled with various stressors, challenges, and responsibilities. In times of difficulty or emotional distress, individuals may turn to pornography as a way to escape from their real-life problems temporarily. Engaging with explicit content can create a distraction, offering a break from daily worries and concerns.

2. Coping Mechanism:

For some people, pornography becomes a coping mechanism to manage stress, anxiety, or negative emotions. When faced with overwhelming emotions, they may seek comfort and relief in the temporary pleasure provided by explicit content. The brief respite it offers can provide a sense of relief and relaxation.

3. Instant Gratification and Pleasure:

Pornography provides instant gratification and pleasure, which can be appealing when individuals seek a quick mood boost or distraction from emotional pain. This immediate reward reinforces the behavior and may lead to using porn as a coping mechanism more frequently.

4. Avoidance of Emotional Processing:

Engaging with explicit content can allow individuals to avoid confronting or processing their emotional issues directly. Rather than dealing with challenging emotions or addressing the root causes of stress, they may turn to pornography as a means of avoiding emotional discomfort.

5. Boredom and Monotony:

In moments of boredom or monotony, individuals may turn to pornography to fill the void and add excitement to their lives. The novelty and variety offered by explicit content can temporarily alleviate feelings of boredom.

It's important to note that while pornography may provide temporary relief or escape, it does not address the underlying issues causing stress or negative emotions. In fact, excessive consumption of pornography as a coping mechanism can lead to a cycle of dependence and further emotional distress in the long run.

Moreover, using pornography as a primary coping strategy can hinder the development of healthy emotional regulation skills and effective problem-solving methods. It may also contribute to a disconnect between an individual's real-life experiences and the unrealistic portrayals often found in porn.

For those who find themselves using pornography as a form of escape or stress relief, seeking healthier alternatives is essential. Engaging in activities that promote relaxation, such as mindfulness exercises, hobbies, physical exercise, or spending time with loved ones, can be more effective in reducing stress and improving emotional well-being in the long term. Counseling or therapy can also be beneficial in developing healthier coping strategies and addressing underlying emotional challenges.

4. Fantasy and Imagination: Pornography caters to fantasies and imaginations, allowing individuals to

explore scenarios and experiences that may not be possible or acceptable in real life.Fantasy and imagination play a significant role in the allure of pornography. Here's a more detailed explanation:

1. Safe Exploration of Desires:

Pornography provides a safe and private space for individuals to explore their sexual desires and fantasies without the need for real-life enactment. People may have fantasies that are considered taboo, unconventional, or even socially unacceptable, but through explicit content, they can indulge in these thoughts without the fear of judgment or consequences.

2. Escaping from Reality:

Explicit content offers an escape from the mundane or stressful aspects of daily life. It allows individuals to temporarily detach from their real-world concerns and immerse themselves in a world of sexual fantasy.

3. Filling the Void of Intimacy:

For some individuals who lack physical intimacy or emotional connection in their lives, pornography may serve as a substitute to temporarily fulfill those needs. It provides a sense of intimacy, even if it is an illusion, and can be comforting in moments of loneliness or isolation.

4. Psychological Comfort:

Fantasies depicted in pornography can offer psychological comfort or reassurance. For example, individuals with body image issues may find reassurance in the diverse representations of bodies in porn, providing a sense of acceptance and validation.

5. Experimentation and Curiosity:

Pornography can satisfy curiosity and encourage sexual experimentation. People may explore new ideas, practices, or roles through explicit content, even if they don't intend to engage in them in real life.

6. Overcoming Inhibition and Anxiety:

For some, pornography can be a way to overcome inhibitions or anxieties related to sexual performance or self-consciousness. It can provide a space to learn about sexual behavior and normalize certain practices.

Potential Pitfalls:

While exploring fantasies through pornography can be a consensual and private activity for some, it is essential to recognize potential pitfalls:

1. Unrealistic Expectations: Pornography often presents idealized and exaggerated portrayals of sex, leading to unrealistic expectations about sexual encounters in real life.
2. Desensitization: Frequent exposure to explicit content can lead to desensitization, making it challenging for individuals to find satisfaction in real-life intimate experiences.
3. Impact on Relationships: The reliance on explicit content to fulfill sexual needs can strain real-life relationships, as it may lead to emotional disconnection and decreased sexual satisfaction with partners.
4. Ethical Concerns: Some pornographic content may exploit or objectify individuals, raising ethical concerns about the industry's practices and potential harm to performers.

While pornography can provide an outlet for exploring fantasies and imagination, it's essential to maintain a critical perspective and approach it with caution. Striking a balance between fantasy and reality, recognizing the limitations of explicit content, and being mindful of its potential impact on mental well-being and relationships is crucial for a healthy approach to sexuality and media consumption. Open communication with partners and a focus on fostering genuine emotional connections can contribute to a more fulfilling and satisfying intimate life.

5. Visual Stimulation: Human brains are highly responsive to visual stimuli. Pornography's explicit and visually appealing nature can trigger arousal and interest.Visual stimulation plays a significant role in human perception and cognition, and the human brain is indeed highly responsive to visual stimuli. Our brains are wired to process visual information efficiently and prioritize it over other sensory inputs. This responsiveness to visuals is a fundamental aspect of human evolution and has important implications for how we engage with the world, including explicit content like pornography.

1. Brain's Visual Processing: The human brain has dedicated areas, such as the occipital lobe at the back of the brain, specifically responsible for visual processing. When we see images or videos, our brains quickly analyze and interpret the visual information, allowing us to understand what we're seeing.

2. Emotional Impact: Visual stimuli can evoke strong emotional responses. The brain's limbic system, which includes structures like the amygdala and hippocampus, plays a role in processing emotions. When we encounter visually appealing or arousing content, it can activate the limbic system, leading to emotional reactions like arousal, excitement, or interest.

3. Immediate Impact: Visual stimuli can have a rapid impact on the brain. Unlike text or other sensory inputs, visual information can be processed quickly, leading to a more immediate response. This quick processing can contribute to the allure of pornography, as it can trigger arousal or interest almost instantly.

4. Attention and Memory: Visually stimulating content tends to capture and hold our attention more effectively than other forms of information. This heightened attention can lead to better memory retention of the visual content, making it more memorable and reinforcing the allure of such stimuli.

5. Evolutionary Significance: The human brain's responsiveness to visual stimuli has evolutionary significance. Throughout human history, the ability to quickly recognize and respond to visual cues has been crucial for survival, such as identifying potential threats, finding food sources, and forming social connections.

6. Media and Advertising: The influence of visual stimuli extends beyond explicit content. It is also exploited in media, advertising, and entertainment industries to engage audiences, promote products, and convey messages effectively.

Regarding pornography, its explicit and visually appealing nature can tap into these inherent neural responses related to visual processing, emotional engagement, and attention. This can lead to the arousal and interest that attracts individuals to consume pornographic content.

However, it's important to note that the allure of pornography should be understood within the broader context of human psychology and individual differences. Not everyone will respond to pornography in the same way, and excessive consumption or addiction can have negative consequences on mental health, relationships, and overall well-being. Responsible consumption, open communication, and awareness of potential impacts are essential when engaging with explicit content.

6. Availability Heuristic: The ready availability of explicit content on the internet reinforces its allure. When something is easily accessible, individuals are more likely to engage with it.The availability heuristic is a cognitive bias that influences how individuals make

decisions and judgments based on the ease with which information comes to mind. In the context of pornography, the availability heuristic plays a significant role in reinforcing its allure due to the easy accessibility of explicit content on the internet.

1. Ease of Access: The internet has revolutionized the way people access information and entertainment, including explicit content. With just a few clicks or taps, individuals can access a vast amount of pornography from the comfort and privacy of their own devices.

2. Constant Presence: Explicit content is pervasive on the internet, and it can be found across various platforms, social media, websites, and streaming services. Its omnipresence increases the likelihood of encountering it during routine internet usage.

3. Minimal Effort Required: Unlike seeking physical media in the past, accessing pornographic content online requires minimal effort or cost. This ease of access removes many barriers that previously limited exposure to explicit content.

4. Reinforcement of Curiosity: The ready availability of pornography fuels curiosity. When individuals become curious about a topic, they are more likely to seek information and explore it further. The internet allows

them to satisfy this curiosity instantaneously, feeding the allure of explicit content.

5. Amplified Social Influence: The internet facilitates social sharing and discussions, and individuals may encounter explicit content through peer recommendations or conversations. Social media platforms, online communities, and chat groups can amplify the availability heuristic by making explicit content a topic of discussion and normalization.

6. Frequent Exposure: The more individuals are exposed to explicit content due to its easy accessibility, the more likely they are to perceive it as a normative or acceptable part of their online experience.

Impact on Behavior:

The availability heuristic can lead individuals to engage with explicit content more frequently than they might have otherwise. The continuous exposure to pornography can reinforce the allure of sexual content, contributing to patterns of excessive consumption and potential addiction.

It's essential to be aware of the influence of the availability heuristic and how it can shape behavior. For parents, educators, and individuals themselves, understanding this cognitive bias can help foster responsible internet usage and informed decision-making regarding explicit content.

Promoting digital literacy and healthy online habits is crucial, especially for young adults, to empower them to navigate the internet responsibly and critically evaluate the information and content they encounter. Encouraging open conversations about the potential consequences of excessive porn consumption can also play a vital role in fostering a balanced approach to sexuality and mental well-being in the digital age.

Neurobiological Aspects:

Dopamine Release: The brain's reward system, centered on the release of dopamine, plays a crucial role. Dopamine is associated with pleasure, motivation, and reinforcement, reinforcing the desire to seek out pornographic content. The Brain's Reward System:

The brain's reward system is a complex network of neural pathways and structures that play a fundamental role in motivating behavior. It is designed to reinforce actions that are essential for survival and well-being, such as eating, drinking, and reproducing. When these actions are performed, the brain releases a neurotransmitter called dopamine.

2. Dopamine: The "Feel-Good" Chemical:
Dopamine is often referred to as the "feel-good" chemical because it contributes to feelings of pleasure, satisfaction, and reward. It acts as a messenger between nerve cells (neurons) in the brain, transmitting signals and facilitating communication.
3. Role of Dopamine in Pleasure and Motivation:
When we engage in activities that are rewarding or pleasurable, such as eating our favorite food or spending time with loved ones, dopamine is released in the brain. This release of dopamine serves as a positive reinforcement, making us more likely to repeat the behavior that led to its release. It helps create a sense of motivation and drives us to seek out experiences that we find enjoyable or rewarding.
4. Dopamine and Pornography:
Pornography can also trigger the release of dopamine in the brain. When individuals view explicit content, the brain perceives it as a rewarding experience, leading to dopamine release. This reinforces the association between viewing pornography and pleasure, creating a desire to seek out more of it.
5. Dopamine and Addiction:
Addictive substances and behaviors, including drugs, alcohol, and certain activities like gambling or gaming, can also trigger the release of dopamine in the brain. In the case of pornography addiction, the repeated release

of dopamine during porn consumption can lead to the reinforcement of the behavior, making it difficult to resist the urge to view more explicit content.

6. Tolerance and Desensitization:

With continued exposure to explicit content, the brain's reward system can undergo changes. Over time, individuals may develop tolerance to the dopamine release, requiring more explicit or novel content to achieve the same level of pleasure. This phenomenon is similar to how drug tolerance develops in substance addiction. Additionally, some individuals may experience desensitization, where the brain becomes less responsive to the usual stimuli, leading to the pursuit of more extreme or novel material to maintain the same level of excitement.

7. Withdrawal and Craving:

When individuals attempt to reduce or quit their porn consumption, they may experience withdrawal symptoms, as mentioned earlier. These symptoms can include intense cravings for pornography, which is a result of the brain's dependence on the dopamine release associated with porn consumption.

Understanding the role of dopamine in the brain's reward system is essential in comprehending the allure of pornography and its potential addictive nature. Responsible use, self-awareness, and seeking support when necessary are essential in promoting a balanced and healthy approach to sexuality and well-being.

Neural Plasticity: The brain's ability to adapt and change, known as neural plasticity, allows it to form new connections based on experiences. Repeated exposure to explicit content can lead to the strengthening of neural pathways associated with the allure of pornography.Neural plasticity, also known as brain plasticity or neuroplasticity, refers to the brain's remarkable ability to adapt and change throughout an individual's life. It involves the formation of new neural connections (synapses) and the reorganization of existing ones in response to experiences, learning, and environmental influences.

Process of Neural Plasticity:

1. Learning and Experience: When we learn new information or engage in various experiences, specific neural pathways in the brain are activated. These pathways consist of interconnected neurons that communicate through chemical and electrical signals.

2. Strengthening Connections: Repeated exposure to a particular experience or behavior strengthens the synaptic connections in the corresponding neural pathways. This process, known as long-term potentiation (LTP), enhances the

communication between neurons involved in the experience.

3. Weakening Connections: Conversely, lack of use or disuse of certain neural pathways weakens the connections through a process called long-term depression (LTD). This allows the brain to adapt and prioritize more relevant connections.

4. Synaptic Pruning: Additionally, neural plasticity involves synaptic pruning, where unnecessary or unused synapses are eliminated. This process streamlines the brain's neural networks, making them more efficient.

Neural Plasticity and Pornography:

When it comes to pornography consumption, neural plasticity plays a significant role in shaping the brain's response to explicit content. Repeated exposure to pornographic material can lead to the following effects:

1. Sensitization: Frequent exposure to explicit content can sensitize certain neural pathways associated with sexual arousal and reward. This can result in a heightened response to pornography, leading to a stronger allure and craving for more explicit material.

2. Desensitization: On the other hand, the brain's reward system can become desensitized to the same level of arousal with repeated exposure to explicit content. As a result, individuals may seek more extreme or novel forms of porn to achieve the same level of pleasure, leading to escalation.

3. Cue Reactivity: Neural plasticity can cause individuals to develop strong responses to environmental cues associated with pornography, such as specific images or contexts. These cues can trigger cravings and compulsive behaviors.

4. Behavior Reinforcement: Neural plasticity reinforces the neural pathways related to engaging with pornographic content, making the behavior more automatic and habitual.

5. Memory Associations: The brain forms associations between pornography and the pleasurable feelings experienced during arousal. These associations can make it challenging for individuals to resist engaging with explicit content, as the brain perceives it as rewarding.

It's important to note that neural plasticity can work both ways. With appropriate interventions, such as reducing exposure to explicit content, seeking therapy, or adopting healthier habits, the brain can gradually rewire itself and weaken the allure of pornography. This underscores the importance of understanding neuroplasticity in addressing pornography addiction and promoting healthy behaviors.

Conditioning: The brain can be conditioned to associate certain stimuli (in this case, pornographic content) with reward and pleasure. Over time, this conditioning can intensify the allure of pornography.Conditioning is a psychological concept that describes the process of learning associations between stimuli and responses. It is a fundamental principle of how our brains form connections based on repeated experiences. In the context of pornography, conditioning plays a significant role in intensifying its allure for some individuals.

Here's a more detailed explanation of conditioning and its role in the allure of pornography:

1. Classical Conditioning:

Classical conditioning, also known as Pavlovian conditioning, was first studied by the Russian physiologist Ivan Pavlov. It involves pairing a neutral stimulus with an unconditioned stimulus to create a conditioned response. In Pavlov's famous experiment, he paired the sound of a bell (neutral stimulus) with the presentation of food (unconditioned stimulus), which led to dogs salivating (conditioned response) in response to the sound of the bell alone after repeated pairings.

2. How it Relates to Pornography:

In the context of pornography, individuals may initially encounter explicit content as a neutral or mildly arousing stimulus. However, when combined with the brain's reward system and the release of dopamine during arousal, the brain forms an association between the explicit content and the pleasurable experience. As individuals repeatedly consume pornography and experience pleasure, this pairing strengthens the connection between the stimuli (pornographic content) and the reward (pleasure).

3. Reinforcement Loop:

The brain's reward system operates on a reinforcement loop. When a behavior is rewarded (e.g., experiencing pleasure from viewing explicit content), it reinforces the likelihood of repeating that behavior in the future. As a result, individuals are more likely to seek out pornography again and again due to the association between the explicit content and the pleasurable experience.

4. Intensification of Allure:

Over time, this conditioning process can intensify the allure of pornography. As the neural connections associated with the allure of explicit content strengthen, individuals may find themselves increasingly drawn to pornographic material, seeking it out more frequently to experience the pleasurable feelings associated with arousal and consumption.

5. Potential for Addiction:

In some cases, the conditioning and reinforcement loop can lead to the development of addiction-like behaviors. The brain's reliance on the pleasurable experience derived from pornography can lead to compulsive consumption, where individuals feel driven to seek out explicit content despite negative consequences in other areas of their lives.

It's important to note that not everyone who views pornography will experience conditioning or addictive behaviors. Individual responses to explicit content can vary widely, and factors such as personal experiences, genetics, and social environment all play roles in shaping one's reactions.

Understanding the process of conditioning helps shed light on why some individuals may become increasingly drawn to pornography and highlights the potential risks of excessive and compulsive consumption. For those concerned about their porn consumption, seeking support from mental health professionals or support groups specializing in sexual addiction can be beneficial in addressing any problematic behaviors and fostering a healthier relationship with explicit content.

Habit Formation: Regular engagement with explicit content can lead to the formation of habits. The more ingrained the habit becomes, the stronger its allure may be.Habit formation in the context of pornography consumption refers to the process by which repeated engagement with explicit content leads to the development of automatic and ingrained behavioral patterns. As individuals continue to consume pornography regularly, their brain becomes conditioned to associate specific cues (such as certain websites, images, or videos) with the reward and pleasure derived from viewing explicit content. This conditioning can create a habitual response, making the allure of pornography even stronger. Here's a more detailed explanation:

1. Cue: In the habit formation process, a cue acts as a trigger that prompts the behavior. In the case of pornography consumption, cues can be various stimuli, such as specific websites, social media platforms, or even emotional states like boredom, stress, or loneliness.

2. Routine: The routine is the habitual behavior triggered by the cue. When individuals encounter the cue associated with porn consumption, they engage in the routine of accessing and viewing explicit content.

3. Reward: The reward is the positive reinforcement individuals receive from engaging in the routine. In the context of pornography, the reward is the pleasure and gratification derived from viewing explicit material.

4. Repetition and Reinforcement: As individuals continue to engage in this cycle of cue-routine-reward, the habit becomes more ingrained in their behavior. Each repetition reinforces the neural pathways associated with the behavior, making the habit stronger and more automatic.

5. Craving and Allure: Over time, the brain's reward system becomes sensitized to the cue, creating a craving for the reward (pleasure from pornography consumption). As the habit becomes more entrenched, the allure of pornography intensifies, and individuals may feel a strong compulsion to engage in the behavior even when they don't consciously want to.

6. Triggers and Environmental Cues: The presence of triggers or environmental cues associated with pornography consumption can activate the habit loop, leading to automatic and unconscious engagement in the behavior.
Breaking the Habit Loop:Breaking the habit loop of pornography consumption can be challenging due to the strong reinforcement and conditioning that have taken place in the brain. However, it is possible with determination and strategies such as:

1. Identifying Triggers: Recognizing the cues that lead to the urge to consume explicit content can help individuals interrupt the habit loop.
2. Creating New Responses: Finding alternative activities or coping strategies to respond to triggers can replace the routine of viewing pornography with healthier behaviors.
3. Building Support Networks: Seeking support from friends, family, or support groups can

provide encouragement and accountability during the process of breaking the habit.
4. Mindfulness and Awareness: Practicing mindfulness can help individuals become more aware of their thoughts and feelings, allowing them to better manage cravings and urges.
5. Professional Help: Seeking help from therapists or counselors who specialize in addiction or compulsive behaviors can provide valuable guidance and support.

Breaking the habit of pornography consumption may take time and effort, but with commitment and the right support, individuals can develop healthier patterns of behavior and improve their overall well-being.

Emotional Regulation: Some individuals may use pornography as a way to regulate emotions or cope with stress, leading to a reinforcing cycle of using it for emotional relief.Emotional regulation refers to the ability to manage and cope with one's emotions effectively. It involves recognizing, understanding, and appropriately responding to emotional experiences. Some individuals may turn to pornography as a coping mechanism to regulate their emotions or alleviate stress. This pattern of behavior can create a reinforcing cycle that perpetuates the use of pornography as a means of emotional relief.

Here's how the cycle of using pornography for emotional regulation typically unfolds:

1. Emotional Distress: When individuals experience negative emotions such as stress, anxiety, loneliness, boredom, or sadness, they may seek ways to escape or alleviate these feelings.

2. Seeking Relief: In search of immediate relief, some individuals turn to pornography. The explicit content can provide a temporary distraction from their emotional distress, offering a momentary escape from reality.

3. Dopamine Release: Engaging with pornography triggers the brain's reward system, leading to the release of dopamine. Dopamine is associated with pleasure and positive reinforcement, which can momentarily alleviate emotional distress and provide a sense of relief or pleasure.

4. Temporary Elevation: While consuming pornography, individuals may experience a temporary elevation in mood, as the brain focuses on the pleasurable experience rather than the source of emotional distress.

5. Reinforcement: The temporary alleviation of emotional distress through pornography can reinforce the behavior. The brain learns that engaging with explicit

content offers a quick and easily accessible way to cope with negative emotions, creating a reinforcing cycle.

6. Escalation: Over time, some individuals may find that they need more explicit or extreme content to achieve the same level of relief, leading to increased consumption and potential addiction.

Consequences and Challenges:

Using pornography as a primary coping mechanism for emotional distress can have several negative consequences:

1. Dependency: Relying on pornography as the primary means of emotional regulation may lead to an unhealthy dependency on explicit content, making it difficult to develop healthier coping strategies.
2. Diminished Coping Skills: Regular use of pornography for emotional relief can impede the development of healthy emotional coping skills, leading to difficulties in effectively managing emotions in real-life situations.
3. Escapism: The reliance on pornography as an escape from emotional distress may prevent individuals from addressing the root causes of

their negative emotions, hindering personal growth and self-awareness.

4. Relationship Strain: As individuals withdraw emotionally into the world of pornography, it can strain intimate relationships, leading to communication breakdowns and decreased emotional intimacy with partners.

Breaking the cycle of using pornography for emotional regulation often requires a multifaceted approach, including:

- Developing healthier coping strategies, such as mindfulness techniques, exercise, hobbies, or seeking support from friends and family.
- Identifying triggers for emotional distress and addressing underlying issues through therapy or counseling.
- Establishing clear boundaries and limiting access to explicit content to reduce dependency.
- Seeking professional help if pornography use becomes compulsive or has a significant impact on mental well-being and relationships.

By addressing the underlying emotional needs and finding healthier ways to cope with stress and negative emotions, individuals can work towards breaking the reinforcing cycle and promoting overall well-being.

It's essential to recognize that while pornography may have its allure for many individuals, its excessive and compulsive consumption can lead to negative consequences, such as addiction, relationship issues, and impacts on mental health. Understanding the psychology and neuroscience behind pornography's allure can aid in promoting awareness, responsible consumption, and maintaining a balanced approach to sexuality and well-being.

The Role of Dopamine and the Brain's Reward System

Dopamine and the brain's reward system play a central role in regulating motivation, pleasure, and reinforcement. Understanding their function is crucial in comprehending various behaviors, including addiction and the allure of certain activities like pornography.

1. Dopamine and Reward System Basics:

Dopamine is a neurotransmitter, a chemical messenger in the brain, that plays a vital role in transmitting signals between neurons. It is involved in several brain functions, but its role in the reward system is particularly significant.Dopamine is a crucial neurotransmitter that serves as a chemical messenger in the brain, transmitting signals between nerve cells or neurons. It belongs to a class of chemicals called catecholamines, which are derived from the amino acid tyrosine. Dopamine plays various roles in the brain, but its involvement in the brain's reward system is of particular importance.

Neurotransmitter Function:

Neurotransmitters are chemicals that facilitate communication between neurons in the brain. When a neuron receives an electrical signal, it releases neurotransmitters into the synapse, which is the small gap between two neurons. These neurotransmitters then bind to specific receptors on the surface of the neighboring neuron, transmitting the signal from one neuron to another.

Role in the Reward System:

Dopamine plays a fundamental role in the brain's reward system, which is a complex network of neural pathways involved in motivation, reinforcement, and pleasure. When we engage in activities that are essential for our survival and well-being, such as eating, drinking, or engaging in sexual activities, the brain's reward system is activated.

Dopamine Release:

During rewarding activities, dopamine is released from certain areas of the brain, such as the ventral tegmental area (VTA) and the nucleus accumbens. This release of dopamine signals to the brain that the activity is pleasurable and beneficial, reinforcing the behavior and encouraging its repetition.

Positive Reinforcement:

Dopamine acts as a form of positive reinforcement, encouraging us to seek out and repeat activities that are essential for our survival and well-being. For example, when we eat something delicious and experience pleasure, dopamine is released, reinforcing the behavior of eating and motivating us to seek food again when hungry.

Motivation and Learning:

Dopamine also plays a role in motivation and learning. When we anticipate a rewarding experience, such as achieving a goal or receiving a reward, dopamine levels increase, motivating us to pursue that goal. Additionally, dopamine is involved in the process of associative learning, where we learn to associate certain cues or actions with pleasurable outcomes.

Role in Addiction:

In cases of addiction, certain drugs or behaviors can lead to an excessive release of dopamine in the brain's reward system. This overstimulation can cause the brain to adapt and become more sensitive to the rewarding effects, leading to the development of addictive patterns. Individuals may engage in compulsive behaviors or seek out substances to repeatedly trigger dopamine release, even at the expense of negative consequences.

Overall, dopamine's role in the brain's reward system is essential for shaping our behaviors and motivations, influencing our responses to pleasurable experiences, and contributing to the formation of habits and addictions. However, maintaining a balanced reward system is crucial for overall well-being and avoiding the potential negative effects of excessive dopamine stimulation.

2. The Brain's Reward System:

The brain's reward system is a complex network of neural pathways that reinforces behaviors that are essential for survival, such as eating, drinking, and reproducing. When these behaviors are carried out, the brain releases dopamine, leading to feelings of pleasure and satisfaction. This positive reinforcement encourages individuals to repeat these behaviors, ensuring the continuity of vital actions.The brain's reward system is an intricate network of neural circuits that evolved to ensure the survival and well-being of organisms. It plays a crucial role in motivating individuals to engage in behaviors necessary for their survival and the continuation of the species. This system is deeply rooted in our evolutionary history and is associated with feelings of pleasure and satisfaction.

Key Components of the Brain's Reward System:

1. Dopamine Pathways:

At the heart of the brain's reward system are dopamine pathways. Dopamine is a neurotransmitter that acts as a chemical messenger, transmitting signals between neurons in the brain. It is released in response to rewarding or pleasurable experiences, promoting positive reinforcement for certain behaviors.

2. Nucleus Accumbens:

The nucleus accumbens is a crucial part of the reward system located in the ventral striatum of the brain. It is often referred to as the brain's pleasure center. When dopamine is released in the nucleus accumbens in response to a rewarding stimulus, it contributes to the feeling of pleasure and reinforces the behavior that led to the reward.

3. Prefrontal Cortex:

The prefrontal cortex, specifically the ventromedial prefrontal cortex, plays a role in decision-making, impulse control, and evaluating the potential rewards and risks associated with certain behaviors. It helps to weigh the benefits and consequences of actions before initiating them.

4. Hippocampus:

The hippocampus is involved in memory formation and learning. It helps to link rewarding experiences with the context in which they occur, contributing to the learning and repetition of behaviors that led to the pleasurable outcomes.

The Process of Positive Reinforcement:

When individuals engage in behaviors essential for their survival or well-being, such as eating, drinking, or reproducing, the brain's reward system is activated:

1. Stimulus and Behavior: When an individual encounters a rewarding stimulus or engages in a behavior linked to survival, such as eating a delicious meal, drinking water when thirsty, or engaging in sexual activity, the brain takes note of this experience.
2. Dopamine Release: In response to the rewarding stimulus or behavior, dopamine is released from the midbrain into the nucleus accumbens and other regions of the brain. This release of

dopamine creates feelings of pleasure and satisfaction, positively reinforcing the behavior.

3. Learning and Repetition: The brain's hippocampus helps to associate the rewarding experience with the specific context and behavior that led to it. This learning process encourages the individual to repeat the behavior in similar situations to attain the reward.

4. Motivation: The positive reinforcement of pleasurable experiences strengthens the individual's motivation to engage in the same behavior again in the future. This motivation ensures the continuity of behaviors necessary for survival and well-being.

Modern Implications:

While the brain's reward system was designed to support essential survival behaviors, modern society offers an abundance of stimuli that can trigger the release of dopamine. This includes not only basic needs like food and water but also various forms of entertainment, social interactions, and addictive substances or behaviors like drugs, gambling, and pornography.

As a result, the brain's reward system can be hijacked by certain activities or substances, leading to addiction and other behavioral issues when individuals become overly reliant on the pleasurable experiences provided by these stimuli.

Understanding the brain's reward system is essential in comprehending human motivation, behavior, and the development of certain psychological disorders. It also sheds light on the allure of activities like pornography, as they can trigger the release of dopamine and create a reinforcing cycle that encourages repeated engagement. By recognizing the power of this system, researchers and clinicians can work toward developing effective strategies for addressing addiction and promoting well-being.

3. Pleasure and Motivation:

Dopamine is often associated with feelings of pleasure and motivation. When an individual engages in activities that the brain perceives as rewarding or pleasurable, such as eating their favorite food or engaging in sexual activities, dopamine is released. This release of dopamine serves as a signal to the brain that the activity is beneficial and should be repeated.Dopamine and Reward Pathway:

Dopamine is a neurotransmitter primarily produced in several areas of the brain, including the ventral tegmental area (VTA) and substantia nigra. One of the brain's major dopamine pathways is the mesolimbic pathway, which connects the VTA to various regions in the brain, including the nucleus accumbens and the prefrontal cortex.

Pleasure and Dopamine Release:

When an individual engages in activities that the brain perceives as pleasurable or rewarding, such as eating delicious food or engaging in sexual activities, dopamine is released from the VTA and travels along the mesolimbic pathway. This dopamine release creates a sensation of pleasure and reinforces the positive feelings associated with the activity.

Motivation and Reinforcement:

Dopamine also plays a key role in motivation and reinforcement. When dopamine is released during a rewarding activity, it acts as a signal to the brain that the behavior is beneficial and should be repeated. This positive reinforcement strengthens the neural connections related to the rewarded behavior, making it more likely that the individual will engage in that activity again in the future.

Learning and Habit Formation:

The brain's reward system is intricately involved in learning and forming habits. As the brain associates certain activities with pleasure and reward due to dopamine release, it becomes more motivated to seek out those activities again. This process facilitates learning and forms habits, shaping an individual's behaviors and preferences.

Addiction and Dopamine:

In the context of addiction, substances or behaviors that lead to an excessive release of dopamine can hijack the brain's reward system. Drugs, for example, can cause a rapid and intense surge of dopamine, creating a powerful reinforcing effect that drives individuals to seek out the substance compulsively. Similarly, addictive behaviors like gambling, gaming, or pornography can trigger dopamine release and lead to repetitive patterns of engagement.

Tolerance and Dopamine Desensitization:

With repeated exposure to rewarding stimuli, the brain can develop a tolerance to the dopamine release. This means that over time, the same level of dopamine release may not produce the same intensity of pleasure. As a result, individuals may seek more significant amounts of the rewarding stimulus to achieve the same level of pleasure or satisfaction. This tolerance and desensitization can contribute to the escalation of addictive behaviors.

Understanding the relationship between dopamine, pleasure, and motivation is crucial for understanding human behavior, addiction, and how the brain's reward system influences our choices and actions. It also highlights the importance of finding a balance in seeking pleasurable activities while avoiding excessive and potentially harmful behaviors that can disrupt overall well-being.

4. Role in Addiction:

Dopamine plays a critical role in addiction. Activities or substances that lead to an excessive release of dopamine can lead to the rewiring of the brain's reward system. In the case of substance addiction, drugs can cause a surge of dopamine, creating a powerful reinforcement of drug-seeking behaviors. Similarly, behaviors like gambling, gaming, or pornography consumption can trigger the release of dopamine, leading to addictive patterns.Dopamine and Reward Processing:

Dopamine is a neurotransmitter that plays a crucial role in the brain's reward processing. When we engage in activities that are pleasurable or rewarding, such as eating delicious food, spending time with loved ones, or achieving a goal, dopamine is released in certain brain regions, such as the nucleus accumbens. This release of dopamine reinforces the behavior, making us more likely to repeat it in the future.

2. Dopamine Release and Addiction:

In the context of addiction, certain substances or behaviors can lead to a rapid and excessive release of dopamine in the brain's reward system. Drugs like cocaine, opioids, or alcohol, as well as addictive behaviors like gambling, gaming, and pornography consumption, can cause a surge of dopamine.

3. Rewiring the Brain's Reward System:

With repeated exposure to these substances or behaviors, the brain's reward system can undergo significant changes. The overstimulation of dopamine receptors can lead to a phenomenon known as neuroplasticity. This is when the brain adapts by forming new connections and altering neural pathways to accommodate the increased dopamine levels.

4. Desensitization and Tolerance:

As the brain's reward system adapts to the increased dopamine levels, it can become desensitized to the same level of stimulation. This can lead to the development of tolerance, where individuals require higher amounts of the substance or behavior to achieve the same level of pleasure they initially experienced.

5. Cravings and Compulsive Behavior:

As the brain's reward system becomes wired to expect the heightened dopamine release from the addictive substance or behavior, cravings can occur. These cravings drive individuals to seek out the addictive stimulus, leading to compulsive behaviors and a loss of control over their actions.

6. Negative Reinforcement:

In addiction, individuals may continue engaging in the addictive behavior or substance use to avoid negative emotions associated with withdrawal. This aspect of addiction is known as negative reinforcement, where the addictive activity serves as a way to escape discomfort or emotional distress.

7. Impaired Decision-Making:

The changes in the brain's reward system can also impact decision-making processes. Individuals with addiction may prioritize seeking out the addictive substance or behavior over other important aspects of their life, leading to negative consequences in relationships, work, and overall well-being.

8. Cycle of Addiction:

The combination of heightened dopamine release, neuroplasticity, tolerance, cravings, and impaired decision-making can perpetuate a cycle of addiction. Individuals become trapped in a pattern where seeking out the addictive substance or behavior becomes the primary focus, despite the negative consequences it may bring.

Understanding the role of dopamine in addiction helps researchers and healthcare professionals develop targeted interventions and treatment strategies for individuals struggling with substance use disorders or behavioral addictions. Treatment often involves addressing both the neurological aspects of addiction and the underlying psychological factors that contribute to its development and maintenance.

5. Tolerance and Desensitization:

Repeated exposure to rewarding stimuli can lead to a process called tolerance, where the brain becomes less responsive to the same level of dopamine release. As a result, individuals may need more significant amounts of the stimulus (e.g., drugs or explicit content) to achieve the same level of pleasure or satisfaction.Tolerance and desensitization are phenomena that occur as a result of repeated exposure to rewarding stimuli, such as drugs, certain behaviors, or explicit content like pornography. These processes can have significant implications for addictive behaviors and the need for increasing amounts of the stimulus to achieve the same level of satisfaction.

Tolerance:

Tolerance refers to the brain's decreasing sensitivity to the effects of a particular stimulus over time. In the context of dopamine and the brain's reward system, this means that with repeated exposure to a rewarding stimulus, the brain becomes less responsive to the dopamine release that the stimulus initially triggered. As a result, the individual may no longer experience the same level of pleasure or satisfaction from the activity or substance as they did during the initial exposures.

Desensitization:

Desensitization, also known as downregulation, is closely related to tolerance. It involves a decrease in the number of dopamine receptors or a reduction in their sensitivity to dopamine. When the brain is consistently flooded with dopamine due to repeated exposure to a rewarding stimulus, it may adjust by reducing the number of available dopamine receptors or making them less responsive to dopamine. This means that the brain becomes less sensitive to the effects of dopamine, leading to reduced pleasure or satisfaction from the stimulus.

Implications for Addiction:

Tolerance and desensitization have significant implications for addiction. As the brain becomes less responsive to the dopamine release from a particular behavior or substance, individuals may seek to compensate by increasing their consumption or engagement. For example:

- In substance addiction, a person may need to take higher doses of a drug to experience the same level of euphoria they once felt with lower amounts.
- In the context of pornography addiction, an individual may need to seek more explicit or

extreme content to achieve the same level of arousal or pleasure they initially experienced with milder content.

The Cycle of Increasing Consumption:

This cycle of increasing consumption is often a hallmark of addiction. As individuals develop tolerance and desensitization to the rewarding stimulus, they may continuously escalate their engagement to chase the initial feelings of pleasure or satisfaction. However, this escalation can have adverse consequences on mental health, relationships, and overall well-being.

Breaking the Cycle:

Breaking the cycle of tolerance and desensitization in addiction often involves reducing or abstaining from the addictive behavior. By doing so, the brain can gradually regain its sensitivity to dopamine, allowing individuals to find pleasure in more moderate and healthier activities.

Seeking professional help, such as therapy or counseling, can be beneficial in addressing addiction and developing healthier coping mechanisms. Therapists can assist individuals in understanding the underlying causes of addiction, providing strategies to manage cravings and withdrawal symptoms, and supporting the journey to recovery and overall well-being.

6. Withdrawal and Cravings:

When the brain's reward system is conditioned to expect the release of dopamine from a particular behavior or substance, the absence of that stimulus can lead to withdrawal symptoms and cravings. For instance, individuals with substance addictions may experience withdrawal symptoms when trying to quit, while those with behavioral addictions like pornography may have strong cravings when attempting to reduce or abstain from engaging in the behavior. Withdrawal and cravings are significant aspects of addiction, whether it involves substances or behavioral addictions like pornography. They occur when an individual's brain has become dependent on a particular behavior or substance to release dopamine, leading to a reinforcing cycle of seeking that stimulus for pleasure and reward.

Withdrawal:

Withdrawal refers to a set of physiological and psychological symptoms that arise when a person reduces or stops engaging in an addictive behavior or discontinues the use of a substance to which they are addicted. These symptoms occur because the brain has become accustomed to the presence of the addictive stimulus and has made adaptations to maintain a state of balance.

In the context of pornography addiction, when an individual attempts to reduce or abstain from consuming explicit content, they may experience withdrawal symptoms such as:

- Intense cravings or urges to view pornography
- Irritability and mood swings
- Anxiety or restlessness
- Difficulty sleeping
- Physical discomfort or restlessness

The severity and duration of withdrawal symptoms can vary based on the individual's level of addiction and their brain's neurochemistry. Withdrawal symptoms can be challenging to endure, leading some individuals to relapse to alleviate the discomfort.

Cravings:

Cravings are intense desires or urges to engage in the addictive behavior or consume the addictive substance.

They arise when the brain's reward system has become conditioned to associate the behavior or substance with the release of dopamine and the subsequent feelings of pleasure and reward.

In the case of pornography addiction, cravings manifest as a strong desire to view explicit content. These cravings can be triggered by various cues, such as stress, boredom, or exposure to certain images or stimuli associated with pornography.

Cravings can be powerful and challenging to resist, as the brain's conditioning reinforces the belief that engaging in the addictive behavior will provide relief and pleasure.

Breaking the Cycle:

Overcoming withdrawal and cravings is a crucial step in recovering from addiction. It requires a combination of strategies, including:

- Support and Accountability: Seeking support from friends, family, or support groups can provide encouragement and accountability during the recovery process.
- Coping Strategies: Developing healthier coping strategies to manage stress, emotions, and

- triggers can help individuals resist the temptation to relapse.
- Professional Help: In some cases, addiction may require professional intervention, such as counseling or therapy, to address underlying issues and develop effective coping mechanisms.
- Avoiding Triggers: Identifying and avoiding triggers that lead to cravings can reduce the likelihood of relapse.
- Self-Reflection: Engaging in self-reflection and understanding the reasons behind the addiction can aid in breaking the reinforcing cycle.

Recovery from addiction is a challenging journey that requires dedication, patience, and a commitment to change. Understanding the role of withdrawal and cravings in addiction can help individuals better navigate the recovery process and build a healthier, more fulfilling life.

7. Balance and Adaptability:

While dopamine is crucial for motivation and reward, maintaining a balance is essential. Overstimulation of the reward system, as seen in addictive behaviors, can lead to adverse consequences on mental and physical health.

The brain's plasticity allows it to adapt to changing circumstances and experiences, which can be both beneficial and detrimental, depending on the context.Dopamine plays a critical role in our daily lives by motivating us to engage in essential activities and reinforcing behaviors that contribute to our survival and well-being. However, maintaining a balance in dopamine activity is crucial for overall mental and physical health. When the brain's reward system is excessively stimulated, as in the case of addictive behaviors, it can lead to detrimental consequences.

1. Addiction and Overstimulation:

In addiction, whether it's substance-related or behavioral (like gambling, gaming, or pornography), the repeated and excessive release of dopamine disrupts the brain's natural balance. The brain becomes hypersensitive to the stimulus, leading individuals to crave and seek out the rewarding behavior or substance compulsively. This can result in a cycle of increasing consumption or engagement, leading to negative outcomes in various aspects of life.

2. Adverse Consequences of Overstimulation:

When the brain's reward system is continually flooded with dopamine, it can lead to various adverse consequences:

- Tolerance: As mentioned earlier, tolerance develops when the brain becomes desensitized to the same level of dopamine release, leading individuals to need higher amounts of the stimulus to achieve the same level of pleasure or satisfaction.
- Withdrawal: The absence of the rewarding stimulus can result in withdrawal symptoms, which can be physically and emotionally distressing. Withdrawal symptoms often lead to cravings and a strong desire to engage in the addictive behavior again.
- Negative Effects on Decision-making: Overstimulation of the reward system can impair rational decision-making, leading individuals to prioritize immediate rewards over long-term well-being. This can contribute to impulsive behaviors and difficulty in breaking the addictive cycle.
- Mental Health Impact: Overstimulation of the reward system has been linked to mental health issues such as depression, anxiety, and other mood disorders.

3. Plasticity and Adaptability of the Brain:

The brain's plasticity, or neuroplasticity, refers to its ability to reorganize and adapt throughout life in response to new experiences and changing circumstances. While plasticity allows the brain to learn, form memories, and recover from injuries, it also means that repeated engagement in certain behaviors can lead to lasting changes in the brain's structure and function.

4. Beneficial and Detrimental Plasticity:

In positive contexts, neuroplasticity enables us to learn new skills, adapt to new environments, and recover from injuries or traumas. However, in negative contexts, such as addiction, plasticity can perpetuate the reinforcing cycle, making it difficult for individuals to break free from the addictive behavior.

5. Rewiring and Habits:

Addictive behaviors can cause the brain to create strong neural pathways associated with the rewarding stimulus, making these behaviors more habitual and challenging to change. Breaking the cycle of addiction often requires forming new, healthier habits and gradually rewiring the brain to prioritize other rewarding activities that contribute to well-being.

While dopamine and the brain's reward system are essential for motivation and reinforcement, maintaining a balance is crucial for overall mental and physical health. Overstimulation of the reward system through addictive behaviors can have adverse consequences. The brain's plasticity allows it to adapt and change, which can be both beneficial and detrimental. Breaking free from addictive behaviors often involves forming healthier habits and gradually rewiring the brain to prioritize activities that promote well-being and balance.

Understanding the role of dopamine and the brain's reward system is vital in comprehending addictive behaviors, the allure of certain activities, and how various external stimuli can impact our mental and emotional well-being.

Chapter 3

The Objectification of Individuals in Pornography

Analyzing the Effects of Objectification on Consumers and Society

The effects of objectification, particularly in the context of media and advertising, can have significant impacts on consumers and society as a whole. Objectification refers to the reduction of a person to the status of an object, emphasizing their physical appearance or sexual appeal over their other qualities and humanity. Here's an analysis of its effects:

Effects on Consumers:

1. Self-Esteem and Body Image: Exposure to objectifying images can negatively impact individuals' self-esteem and body image. Constant exposure to unrealistic beauty standards can lead to feelings of inadequacy and dissatisfaction with one's own appearance.
2. Psychological Well-being: Objectification can contribute to increased levels of anxiety, depression, and stress. Individuals may feel pressured to conform to societal beauty norms, causing emotional distress and reduced well-being.
3. Hypersexualization: Objectification can contribute to the hypersexualization of individuals, particularly women, in media and advertising. This can lead to the perception that a person's worth is tied to their sexual attractiveness, reinforcing harmful gender stereotypes.
4. Relationships: Objectification can impact interpersonal relationships, as individuals may prioritize physical appearance over other qualities when evaluating potential partners. This can lead to shallow or superficial relationships.
5. Sexual Objectification: Objectification can lead to the perception of individuals as mere sexual objects, disregarding their thoughts, feelings, and

autonomy. This dehumanization can increase the risk of sexual harassment, assault, and violence.

Effects on Society:

1. Gender Inequality: Objectification perpetuates gender inequality by reinforcing traditional gender roles and stereotypes. Women, in particular, are often portrayed as objects of desire rather than fully realized individuals with diverse talents and abilities.
2. Normalization of Objectification: Constant exposure to objectifying images in media and advertising can normalize and reinforce objectification in society, leading to its acceptance as a societal norm.
3. Cultural Attitudes: Objectification can influence cultural attitudes toward women and men, shaping how they are perceived and treated in various contexts.
4. Media and Advertising Impact: Objectification in media and advertising can contribute to a toxic culture that prioritizes physical appearance over substance, potentially hindering the representation and recognition of individuals based on their skills and achievements.

5. Influence on Children and Adolescents: Exposure to objectifying content can shape the attitudes and beliefs of young people, affecting their self-image, attitudes toward others, and future behavior.

Addressing Objectification:

Addressing the effects of objectification requires collective efforts from various stakeholders:

1. Media and Advertising Industry: Promote responsible portrayal of individuals, avoiding objectification and promoting diverse representations that reflect real people's talents and contributions.
2. Education and Awareness: Increase awareness about the harmful effects of objectification through educational programs and campaigns.
3. Regulation: Implement regulations that curb the use of objectifying imagery and promote positive representation in media and advertising.
4. Promote Empowerment: Encourage body positivity and self-acceptance, emphasizing that individuals' worth goes beyond their physical appearance.

5. Media Literacy: Enhance media literacy among consumers to help them critically analyze and resist objectifying messages.

By addressing the effects of objectification on consumers and society, we can work towards creating a more inclusive, respectful, and empowering environment that values individuals for their true worth and humanity rather than reducing them to mere objects.

Navigating the Thin Line Between Fantasy and Reality

Navigating the thin line between fantasy and reality is essential to maintaining a healthy and balanced perspective on life. While fantasies can be a natural and harmless part of the human imagination, it is crucial to distinguish them from reality to avoid potential negative consequences. Here are some key points to consider:

1. Understanding Fantasy:

Fantasies are imaginative thoughts, desires, or scenarios that are not based in reality. They can be about various aspects of life, such as romantic relationships, career aspirations, or personal achievements. Fantasies can provide an escape from everyday life or serve as a source of inspiration.

2. Differentiating Fantasy from Reality:

It's essential to recognize the boundary between fantasy and reality. While fantasies can be enjoyable and entertaining, they should not be mistaken for achievable or realistic goals. Distinguishing between what is possible and what is purely a product of imagination helps maintain a grounded perspective.

3. Managing Expectations:

Understanding the difference between fantasy and reality is crucial for managing expectations in various areas of life. Setting realistic goals and expectations based on real-world possibilities can prevent disappointment and frustration.

4. Impact on Relationships:

In romantic relationships, it's important to recognize that fantasies about an ideal partner or relationship may not align with reality. Unrealistic expectations can strain relationships and hinder genuine emotional connections.

5. Escapism vs. Avoidance:

While occasional daydreaming and fantasizing can be healthy forms of escapism, relying too heavily on fantasies to avoid real-life challenges or problems can be detrimental. Addressing real issues and finding practical solutions is essential for personal growth and well-being.

6. Responsible Media Consumption:

Media, including movies, TV shows, books, and online content, often portray fantastical scenarios. Enjoying these forms of entertainment is fine, but being aware of their fictional nature is crucial to avoid confusing them with reality.

7. Balanced Self-Expression:

Fantasies can inspire creativity and self-expression. It's important to find healthy outlets for creative expression while understanding the boundary between imaginative creations and real-life actions.

8. Cultivating Mindfulness:

Practicing mindfulness can help bring awareness to the present moment and distinguish between fantasy and reality. Mindfulness allows individuals to observe their thoughts without judgment, helping them stay grounded in the present.

9. Seeking Professional Help:

In some cases, individuals may struggle with differentiating between fantasy and reality due to mental health issues. Seeking guidance from mental health professionals can be beneficial in addressing such challenges.

By being mindful of the thin line between fantasy and reality, individuals can enjoy the benefits of creative imagination while remaining grounded in the present and making informed decisions about their lives. Striking this balance contributes to overall well-being and healthier relationships with oneself and others.

Chapter 4

The Journey of Healing and Recovery

Recognizing the Signs of Porn Addiction in Young Adults

Recognizing the signs of porn addiction in young adults can be challenging, as some behaviors might be mistaken for normal curiosity or experimentation. However, it's essential to be vigilant and aware of potential red flags that may indicate a problem. Here are some signs to look out for:

Compulsive Behavior: Young adults addicted to porn may engage in the habit compulsively, spending excessive time consuming explicit content, even when it interferes with other essential activities or responsibilities.Compulsive behavior refers to the repetitive engagement in an activity despite negative consequences or a desire to stop. In the context of porn addiction, young adults may exhibit compulsive behaviors related to consuming explicit content online. Here are some key aspects of compulsive behavior in relation to porn addiction:

Frequent and Prolonged Consumption: Young adults addicted to porn may spend a significant amount of time watching explicit content, often for hours at a time. They may struggle to control the duration of their consumption, leading to excessive viewing sessions that interfere with other aspects of their lives.

Neglecting Responsibilities: As porn consumption takes precedence, young adults may neglect their responsibilities at school, work, or home. This can lead to declining academic or job performance and increased conflict with family members or roommates.

Inability to Stop: Despite recognizing the negative consequences of their porn consumption, individuals with addiction may find it difficult to stop or cut back on their habits. The pull of the habit becomes overwhelming, and the desire to engage in other activities diminishes.

Preoccupation and Cravings: Young adults addicted to porn may constantly think about the next opportunity to watch explicit content, experiencing strong cravings that distract them from their daily tasks and activities.

Escalation of Consumption: Over time, individuals with porn addiction may find that they need more explicit or extreme content to achieve the same level of pleasure. This escalation can lead to exploring more graphic or niche genres to satisfy their cravings.

Sense of Loss of Control: Addiction can leave young adults feeling powerless over their behavior. They may feel trapped in a cycle of consumption, wanting to stop but unable to do so without outside help or intervention.

Negative Impact on Well-Being: Compulsive porn consumption can negatively impact mental and emotional well-being. Individuals may experience guilt, shame, or low self-esteem as a result of their addiction.

It's crucial to approach the topic of porn addiction with empathy and understanding. Addiction is a complex issue that often involves underlying emotional, psychological, or environmental factors. If you suspect that a young adult is struggling with porn addiction, offering support and encouragement to seek professional help can make a significant difference in their journey toward recovery and well-being. Remember that seeking help from qualified therapists or support groups specializing in sexual addiction is essential for addressing the issue effectively.

Increased Isolation: Porn addiction can lead to social withdrawal. Young adults may prefer spending time alone to engage in their habit rather than interacting with friends or family.One of the signs of porn addiction in young adults is a noticeable increase in isolation. As their consumption of explicit content intensifies, they may withdraw from social interactions and prefer spending more time alone to engage in their habit. This isolation can manifest in various ways:

A. Avoiding Social Activities: Young adults addicted to porn may start avoiding social gatherings, parties, or outings with friends and family. They might decline invitations or make excuses to spend more time alone, creating distance from their social circles.

B. Reduced Communication: Addicted individuals may become less communicative and responsive to friends and family. They may withdraw emotionally, becoming less engaged in conversations and interactions with loved ones.

C. Prioritizing Privacy: To indulge in their porn consumption without interference, addicted young adults might actively seek out opportunities for privacy. They may spend more time in their rooms or lock themselves in private spaces to avoid being discovered.

D. Decreased Interest in Hobbies and Activities: As porn consumption takes up more of their time and attention, young adults may lose interest in activities they once enjoyed. They might abandon hobbies, sports, or other extracurricular pursuits in favor of spending time alone with explicit content.

E. Digital Disconnection: Young adults addicted to porn may become increasingly absorbed in their online activities, reducing interaction with friends on social media and other digital platforms.

Possible Causes of Increased Isolation:

Several factors can contribute to the increased isolation observed in young adults struggling with porn addiction:

1. Shame and Guilt: Feelings of shame and guilt associated with porn consumption can lead to self-imposed isolation as individuals try to hide their habit from others.
2. Escapism: Porn consumption may serve as a form of escape from real-life challenges and emotions, prompting young adults to seek solitude as they engage in this habit.
3. Social Stigma: Young adults may be aware of the social stigma surrounding pornography consumption, leading them to withdraw from social interactions to avoid judgment or criticism.
4. Preoccupation: The addictive nature of porn can preoccupy individuals' thoughts and time, leaving little mental or emotional space for maintaining social connections.

Addressing Increased Isolation:

If you observe increased isolation in a young adult, it's essential to approach the situation with empathy and understanding. Engaging in open and non-judgmental communication can help create a safe space for the individual to share their experiences and concerns.

Encouraging them to seek professional help from therapists or support groups specializing in sexual addiction can be beneficial. By addressing the underlying issues and providing support, young adults can gradually work towards reconnecting with their social circles and finding healthier ways to cope with stress and emotions. Building a supportive network can play a crucial role in their journey towards recovery and overall well-being.

Neglecting Relationships: A significant sign of porn addiction is neglecting real-life relationships in favor of consuming explicit content. This can lead to a decline in social and emotional connections with friends, family, or romantic partners.Porn addiction can significantly impact a young adult's ability to maintain healthy and meaningful relationships with others. As their addiction intensifies, they may become increasingly preoccupied with consuming explicit content, leading to the neglect of their real-life relationships. Here are some key points to consider:

1. Social Withdrawal: Young adults struggling with porn addiction may withdraw socially to engage in their habit in privacy. They might avoid social gatherings, outings with friends, or family events to have more time for consuming explicit content.

2. Emotional Disconnection: Addiction to pornography can lead to emotional disconnection from loved ones. The excessive focus on explicit content might prevent them from fully engaging emotionally with their friends, family, or romantic partners.

3. Decline in Intimacy: Porn addiction can adversely affect romantic relationships, leading to a decline in intimacy and emotional connection with their partners. The unrealistic nature of explicit content can create unrealistic expectations, making it challenging to maintain genuine and intimate connections.

4. Lack of Communication: Young adults consumed by porn addiction may avoid open communication with others about their struggles. They might fear judgment or criticism, leading to a breakdown in effective communication within relationships.

5. Isolation and Secrecy: They may feel a need to hide their addiction from others, leading to increased isolation and secretive behavior. This isolation can create a divide between them and their loved ones, making it difficult for family and friends to provide support.

6. Emotional Toll on Loved Ones: The neglect of relationships due to porn addiction can have a profound emotional impact on their loved ones. Partners, parents, or close friends may feel hurt, neglected, or unimportant, leading to strain and conflict in the relationship.

7. Escalation of Addiction: As the addiction progresses, individuals may become increasingly consumed by the habit, further isolating themselves and deepening the neglect of their relationships.

It's essential to approach the issue with empathy and understanding. Addiction is a complex challenge, and individuals struggling with porn addiction may feel ashamed or embarrassed to seek help. Creating a supportive and non-judgmental environment can encourage open communication and foster the willingness to address the issue.

If you notice signs of neglecting relationships in a young adult, consider initiating a caring and compassionate conversation. Encourage them to seek professional help from therapists or support groups specializing in sexual addiction. Early intervention and support can help them navigate the challenges of porn addiction, rebuild their relationships, and work towards improved emotional well-being.

Decline in Academic or Job Performance: Porn addiction can impact young adults' ability to focus and concentrate on their studies or work, leading to a decline in academic or job performance.One of the signs of porn addiction in young adults is a decline in academic or job performance. As the addiction takes a toll on their lives, it can interfere with their ability to focus on important tasks related to their education or work. Here's a more detailed explanation of how porn addiction can impact academic or job performance:

1. Lack of Focus and Concentration:

Porn addiction can consume a significant amount of a young adult's time and attention. Constant thoughts about accessing explicit content or planning when and where to view it can lead to a lack of focus and concentration on academic or work-related tasks. This can result in decreased productivity and performance.

2. Procrastination and Time Mismanagement:
When porn becomes an addiction, young adults may prioritize viewing explicit content over their academic or job responsibilities. This can lead to procrastination and poor time management, as they may spend more time indulging in their habit instead of completing important tasks.

3. Reduced Energy and Motivation:
Excessive consumption of pornography can be mentally and emotionally draining. Young adults may experience reduced energy levels and motivation to engage in their studies or job duties.

4. Emotional Distress and Guilt:
Porn addiction can lead to feelings of guilt, shame, or emotional distress. These negative emotions can further hinder academic or job performance, as the young adult may struggle to focus on their responsibilities while dealing with the psychological effects of addiction.

5. Absenteeism or Tardiness:

In severe cases, porn addiction can lead to absenteeism or frequent tardiness. Young adults may skip classes or call in sick to work to engage in their habit, leading to a decline in their attendance and reliability.

6. Impact on Relationships:Struggles with porn addiction can impact relationships with peers, colleagues, or supervisors. The decline in academic or job performance may be noticed by others, potentially leading to strained interpersonal dynamics.

7. Negative Feedback or Disciplinary Actions: A decline in academic or job performance can lead to negative feedback from teachers, professors, supervisors, or co-workers. In academic settings, poor grades or missed deadlines can result in academic probation or disciplinary actions.

8. Loss of Interest or Ambition: Porn addiction can diminish a young adult's interest in their academic pursuits or career goals. The addiction may become the primary focus of their life, overshadowing their aspirations and ambition.

It's important to approach this issue with empathy and understanding. If you notice a young adult experiencing a decline in academic or job performance, it may be beneficial to initiate an open and non-judgmental conversation. Encourage them to seek professional help, such as therapy or counseling, to address the underlying issues related to their porn addiction and academic/work challenges. Early intervention and support can play a crucial role in helping them regain focus, motivation, and a healthier balance in their life.

Escalation of Content: Over time, individuals addicted to porn may seek more explicit or extreme content to achieve the same level of pleasure or excitement, leading to a progression in the type of material they consume.Escalation of content is a characteristic feature of porn addiction, where individuals find themselves seeking more explicit or extreme material to achieve the same level of pleasure or excitement they experienced initially. As the addiction progresses, the content that once satisfied them may no longer have the same impact, leading them to explore increasingly graphic or novel forms of explicit material.

How Escalation Occurs:

Porn addiction can cause changes in the brain's reward system and dopamine pathways. Initially, when individuals engage in explicit content, the brain releases dopamine, resulting in a pleasurable and reinforcing experience. Over time, the brain can become desensitized to the same level of dopamine release, leading to tolerance.

As a result of tolerance, individuals may need more stimulating or explicit content to achieve the same level of pleasure they once experienced. This process of escalating the intensity or graphic nature of pornographic material is a way for the brain to counteract the diminishing pleasure response caused by tolerance.

Potential Consequences:

Escalation of content can have several potential consequences:

1. Normalizing Extreme Content: Over time, individuals may become desensitized to extreme or violent content, leading to a normalization of harmful or abusive material. This can have concerning implications for their attitudes and behaviors in real-life relationships.
2. Influence on Sexual Preferences: Consistent exposure to specific explicit content can influence an individual's sexual preferences and

fantasies, which may deviate from their real-life desires or values.

3. Impact on Relationships: Escalation of content can negatively impact intimate relationships, as the individual may become more focused on fantasy-driven sexual experiences rather than developing genuine emotional connections with their partner.

4. Mental Health Impact: Escalation of content may exacerbate feelings of guilt, shame, or anxiety related to the consumption of explicit material. It can also contribute to emotional distress and hinder overall mental well-being.

Addressing Escalation:

Recognizing the escalation of content is crucial in identifying problematic porn consumption. Addressing the issue requires acknowledging the addictive nature of the behavior and seeking support to break free from the cycle.

Individuals struggling with porn addiction may benefit from:

1. Seeking Professional Help: Talking to a therapist or counselor who specializes in sexual addiction can provide valuable guidance and support.
2. Creating a Support System: Engaging with supportive friends, family, or support groups can be instrumental in overcoming addiction.
3. Using Accountability Tools: Employing accountability software or apps that monitor internet usage can help individuals stay on track with their recovery.
4. Building Healthy Coping Strategies: Finding alternative ways to cope with stress, anxiety, or emotional distress can reduce the reliance on explicit content as a coping mechanism.

Breaking the cycle of escalation and seeking help early on is essential to preventing further negative consequences and promoting healthier patterns of behavior and relationships.

Withdrawal Symptoms: Young adults addicted to porn may experience withdrawal-like symptoms when attempting to reduce or stop their consumption. These symptoms can be emotional, psychological, or even physical in nature.Withdrawal symptoms are a set of physiological and psychological reactions that individuals may experience when they attempt to reduce or stop their porn consumption. Similar to withdrawal symptoms associated with substance addictions, individuals with porn addiction may go through a period of discomfort and distress when trying to abstain from engaging in the habit.

Examples of Withdrawal Symptoms in Porn Addiction:

1. Cravings: Individuals addicted to porn may experience intense cravings or urges to watch explicit content when they try to quit. These cravings can be challenging to resist and may lead to relapses.
2. Irritability and Anxiety: During withdrawal, individuals may feel irritable, anxious, or restless. The absence of the behavior they have grown accustomed to can cause emotional discomfort.
3. Mood Swings: Abruptly stopping porn consumption may lead to mood swings, with individuals experiencing sudden shifts in emotions from sadness to anger or frustration.
4. Insomnia or Sleep Disturbances: Some individuals may have difficulty falling asleep or experience disrupted sleep patterns during withdrawal.

5. Physical Discomfort: In some cases, individuals may experience physical discomfort such as headaches or body aches when trying to abstain from porn consumption.
6. Difficulty Concentrating: Withdrawal can impair concentration and focus, making it challenging for individuals to engage in other activities or responsibilities.
7. Social Withdrawal: During withdrawal, individuals may isolate themselves from others, preferring to be alone rather than facing the discomfort of abstaining from porn.

Duration of Withdrawal Symptoms:

The duration and intensity of withdrawal symptoms can vary depending on the individual and the extent of their addiction. Withdrawal symptoms may last for several days to a few weeks, and in some cases, longer. The initial period of withdrawal can be the most challenging, but with time and support, symptoms tend to subside.

Coping with Withdrawal Symptoms:

Coping with withdrawal symptoms requires determination, support, and healthy coping strategies. Here are some ways individuals can navigate through this challenging phase:

1. Seeking Support: Having a supportive network of friends, family, or professionals can make the withdrawal process more manageable. Talking about the challenges and feelings with a trusted person can provide emotional support.
2. Engaging in Healthy Distractions: Finding alternative activities or hobbies to replace the time spent on porn consumption can be helpful in reducing cravings and staying occupied.
3. Mindfulness and Relaxation Techniques: Practicing mindfulness and relaxation exercises can help individuals manage stress and anxiety during withdrawal.
4. Setting Realistic Goals: Taking small steps and setting realistic goals for reducing porn consumption can make the process more achievable.
5. Avoiding Triggers: Identifying and avoiding triggers that may lead to cravings can help prevent relapses.
6. Professional Help: If withdrawal symptoms are severe or unmanageable, seeking help from therapists or support groups specializing in sexual addiction can be beneficial.

It's important to emphasize that seeking professional help is essential if individuals find it challenging to cope with withdrawal symptoms or if porn addiction is significantly impacting their daily life and well-being. Early intervention and support can make a positive difference in overcoming addiction and improving overall mental health.

1. Secretive Behavior: Individuals struggling with porn addiction may become secretive about their online activities, clearing browsing histories, or using private browsing modes to hide their habits.
2. Impact on Mental Health: Porn addiction can have negative effects on mental health, leading to feelings of guilt, shame, or anxiety related to the habit.
3. Decline in Physical Health: Consuming explicit content for extended periods can lead to physical issues like fatigue, disrupted sleep patterns, or changes in sexual behavior.
4. Attempts to Quit Unsuccessfully: Young adults with porn addiction may try to quit or reduce their consumption but find it challenging to do so, experiencing strong urges or relapsing into old habits.

It's important to remember that the presence of one or two signs does not necessarily indicate porn addiction.

However, if you notice multiple signs or a pattern of problematic behavior, it may be worth having an open and non-judgmental conversation with the young adult to understand their experiences and offer support.

If you suspect that a young adult may be struggling with porn addiction, it's essential to encourage them to seek professional help from therapists or support groups specializing in sexual addiction. Early intervention and support can be crucial in addressing the issue and promoting overall well-being.

Strategies for Breaking Free from Pornography's Grip

Breaking free from pornography's grip can be a challenging but empowering journey. Implementing effective strategies and seeking support can make the process more manageable. Here are some strategies to help individuals overcome pornography addiction:

1. Acknowledge the Issue: The first step is acknowledging that there is a problem and accepting that pornography has a negative impact on your life. Recognizing the addiction is essential for taking action to break free.Acknowledging the issue of pornography addiction is a critical first step towards recovery. It involves recognizing and accepting that consuming explicit content has become a problematic behavior that negatively affects various aspects of your life. Acknowledgment is essential for several reasons:

Self-Awareness: Acknowledging the addiction requires self-awareness and honest self-reflection. It involves understanding the impact of pornography on your emotions, relationships, and overall well-being.

Breaking Denial: Addiction often comes with denial, where individuals may rationalize or minimize the negative consequences of their behavior. Acknowledging the issue breaks through this denial, allowing you to confront the reality of the addiction.

Motivation for Change: Accepting the presence of the addiction provides a powerful incentive to make positive changes in your life. It serves as a starting point for taking responsibility and committing to a healthier path.

Reducing Guilt and Shame: Acknowledgment can help reduce feelings of guilt and shame associated with the addiction. Instead of being trapped in negative emotions, you can focus on moving forward and making improvements.

Openness to Help: Being honest about your struggle with pornography addiction opens the door to seeking support from others. It allows you to reach out to friends, family, or professionals who can offer guidance and understanding.

Steps for Acknowledgment:

Recognizing and accepting pornography addiction requires courage and a willingness to confront difficult emotions. Here are some steps to help you acknowledge the issue:

1. Reflect on the Impact: Take time to honestly assess how pornography consumption has affected your life, relationships, emotions, and overall well-being. Consider the negative consequences and how they align with your values and goals.

2. Identify Patterns: Identify patterns of behavior related to pornography consumption, such as times of day when you are more likely to engage in the habit or specific triggers that prompt the behavior.

3. Seek Feedback: Talk to a trusted friend, family member, or therapist about your struggle with pornography addiction. Their perspective and support can provide valuable insight and encouragement.

4. Avoid Self-Judgment: Acknowledging an addiction can be challenging, and it's normal to have mixed emotions. Avoid self-judgment and recognize that you are taking a brave step towards positive change.

5. Set Realistic Expectations: Recovery is a process, and change takes time. Set realistic expectations for yourself and be patient as you work towards breaking free from pornography's grip.

Remember that acknowledging the issue is only the beginning of the journey towards recovery. The road ahead may have challenges, but acknowledging the addiction empowers you to take control and make the necessary changes to live a healthier, more fulfilling life.

2. Set Clear Goals: Define your goals for reducing or eliminating pornography consumption. Setting specific and achievable goals can provide direction and motivation throughout the recovery process.Why Clear Goals are Important:

Setting clear and specific goals is a crucial step in overcoming pornography addiction for several reasons:

1. Motivation: Clear goals provide motivation and a sense of purpose. When individuals have a clear vision of what they want to achieve, they are more likely to stay committed to the recovery process, even during challenging times.

2. Focus: Defined goals help individuals stay focused on what they want to accomplish. In the context of overcoming addiction, having a clear goal can help individuals redirect their attention and energy away from pornography and toward healthier activities.

3. Measure Progress: Specific goals enable individuals to measure their progress. Tracking progress can be

encouraging and rewarding, as individuals can see their accomplishments over time.

4. Accountability: Setting clear goals can create a sense of accountability. By sharing their goals with a support system or therapist, individuals may feel more responsible for their actions and progress.

5. Identify Obstacles: Having clear goals allows individuals to identify potential obstacles or challenges that may hinder their recovery. By recognizing these obstacles in advance, individuals can develop strategies to overcome them.

Tips for Setting Clear Goals:

1. Be Specific: Clearly define what you want to achieve. For example, a specific goal could be to abstain from pornography for a certain number of days or to reduce consumption to a specific frequency.

2. Make Goals Realistic and Achievable: Set goals that are realistic and achievable within your current circumstances. Setting overly ambitious goals can lead to frustration and demotivation if they are not attainable.

3. Break Goals into Smaller Steps: Breaking larger goals into smaller, manageable steps can make the process feel

less overwhelming. Achieving these smaller milestones can provide a sense of accomplishment and keep you motivated.

4. Write Down Your Goals: Putting your goals in writing can make them more tangible and help reinforce your commitment to achieving them.

5. Establish a Timeline: Set a timeframe for achieving your goals. This timeline should be reasonable and considerate of your individual progress.

6. Review and Adjust Goals: Periodically review your goals and assess your progress. Be open to adjusting your goals if needed, depending on your experiences and developments in your recovery journey.

7. Celebrate Achievements: Celebrate each milestone and achievement along the way. Recognizing your progress can boost your confidence and reinforce your commitment to breaking free from pornography addiction.

Remember, breaking free from pornography addiction is a process that requires dedication and perseverance. Setting clear and meaningful goals can provide a roadmap for your recovery journey and help you reclaim control over your life and well-being. Seek support from loved ones or professionals if needed, and don't hesitate to celebrate your progress along the way.

3. Create a Support System: Reach out to friends, family members, or support groups to share your struggles and seek encouragement. Having a support system can provide understanding, empathy, and accountability.Overcoming pornography addiction can be a challenging and emotional journey. Creating a support system of understanding and caring individuals can be instrumental in providing encouragement, accountability, and motivation throughout the recovery process. Here's why having a support system is crucial:

1. Understanding and Empathy: Addiction can be isolating, and individuals struggling with pornography addiction may feel ashamed or hesitant to discuss their struggles with others. Having a support system allows them to confide in understanding and empathetic individuals who won't judge or criticize them.

2. Non-Judgmental Environment: A supportive network provides a non-judgmental environment where individuals can share their experiences, emotions, and challenges openly. This can create a sense of safety and trust, essential for healing and growth.

3. Accountability: A support system can serve as an accountability mechanism. Sharing your recovery goals with others means that you're more likely to stay committed and motivated to achieve them.

4. Encouragement and Motivation: Supportive friends, family, or support groups can offer encouragement, uplifting words, and motivation during difficult moments. Their belief in your ability to change and overcome the addiction can be a powerful source of inspiration.

5. Share Coping Strategies: Being part of a support system provides an opportunity to learn from others who may have successfully overcome similar challenges. Members can share coping strategies and insights that have worked for them, which can be valuable in developing your own approach to recovery.

6. Preventing Relapses: During the recovery journey, individuals may face triggers or moments of vulnerability that could lead to relapse. A support system can help identify these triggers and provide timely intervention and support to prevent setbacks.

7. Reducing Feelings of Isolation: Knowing that you are not alone in your struggle can significantly reduce feelings of isolation and helplessness. Being part of a

support system reinforces the idea that others understand and stand with you on your journey.

8. Celebrating Milestones: Celebrating milestones and progress with a support system can reinforce positive behaviors and create a sense of achievement, boosting self-confidence.

9. Professional Support Recommendations: Members of a support system may suggest seeking professional help or offer guidance on finding therapists or counselors specialized in sexual addiction when needed.

Types of Support System:

- Family and Friends: Close family members and friends who are empathetic and non-judgmental can form a core support system.
- Support Groups: Joining support groups specifically focused on pornography addiction can provide a community of individuals facing similar challenges.
- Therapists or Counselors: Seeking professional help from therapists or counselors experienced in sexual addiction can offer personalized support and guidance.

- Online Forums and Communities: Online forums or virtual support communities can be beneficial for connecting with others who understand the struggles of addiction.

Creating a support system is a crucial aspect of overcoming pornography addiction. Having understanding, non-judgmental individuals by your side can provide the encouragement, accountability, and motivation needed to navigate the challenges of recovery successfully. Whether it's family, friends, support groups, or professional therapists, the power of a supportive network can significantly contribute to healing and building a healthier future.

4. Educate Yourself: Learn about the harmful effects of pornography addiction to reinforce your commitment to break free from its grip. Understanding the psychological, emotional, and relationship consequences can serve as a powerful motivator.Understanding the Impact: One of the crucial steps in breaking free from pornography's grip is educating oneself about the harmful effects of addiction. Gaining a comprehensive understanding of the psychological, emotional, and relationship consequences of pornography consumption can serve as a powerful motivator to change.

1. Psychological Effects: Regular and excessive consumption of pornography can lead to changes in brain activity, affecting the brain's reward system and dopamine release. This can create an addictive pattern, making it challenging to control the impulse to consume explicit content.

2. Emotional Consequences: Pornography addiction can lead to feelings of guilt, shame, and self-loathing. Individuals may experience a discrepancy between their real-life values and their porn consumption, leading to internal conflicts and emotional distress.

3. Relationship Impact: Pornography addiction can negatively affect intimate relationships. It may lead to decreased emotional intimacy, unrealistic expectations about sex and relationships, and difficulties in establishing trust with partners.

4. Escalation and Desensitization: Over time, some individuals may find that they need more explicit or extreme content to achieve the same level of arousal. This escalation can lead to desensitization, where real-life sexual experiences no longer provide satisfaction.

5. Distorted Perception of Sexuality: Consuming pornography regularly can lead to a distorted perception

of sexuality, often portraying unrealistic and potentially harmful representations of intimate relationships.

6. Objectification and Gender Issues: Frequent exposure to objectifying content in pornography can contribute to the objectification of individuals, particularly women, in real life. This can perpetuate harmful gender stereotypes and contribute to gender inequality.

7. Impact on Mental Health: Pornography addiction has been linked to various mental health issues, including anxiety, depression, and social isolation. It can become a coping mechanism for emotional distress, creating a cycle that further exacerbates mental health challenges.

Empowerment through Knowledge:

Educating oneself about the negative consequences of pornography addiction empowers individuals to make informed decisions about their behavior. Knowledge helps individuals realize that pornography does not represent healthy, authentic intimacy and that there are healthier ways to navigate their sexuality.

Building Motivation and Commitment:

Understanding the damaging effects of pornography addiction can fuel motivation to change. As individuals grasp the impact it has on their well-being and relationships, they may become more committed to breaking free from the addiction.

Supporting Long-Term Recovery:

Education plays a crucial role in long-term recovery. Being aware of the potential consequences of returning to old habits can serve as a deterrent, supporting individuals in their commitment to remain porn-free.

It's important to note that education should be part of a comprehensive approach to overcoming pornography addiction. Combining knowledge with other strategies such as seeking support, developing healthier coping mechanisms, and setting clear goals can maximize the chances of success in breaking free from pornography's grip.

5. Identify Triggers: Identify the situations, emotions, or thoughts that trigger the urge to consume pornography. Recognizing these triggers allows you to develop strategies to avoid or cope with them effectively.Identifying triggers is a crucial step in breaking free from pornography addiction. Triggers are specific situations, emotions, or thoughts that prompt the urge or desire to consume explicit content. By recognizing these triggers, individuals can develop

strategies to avoid or cope with them effectively, reducing the likelihood of engaging in addictive behaviors. Here's a more detailed explanation:

1. Types of Triggers:

Situational Triggers: These are specific circumstances or environments that can lead to the urge to consume pornography. For example, being alone in a private space, having access to the internet or explicit content, or encountering specific places associated with past porn consumption can be situational triggers.

Emotional Triggers: Certain emotions can trigger the desire to use pornography as a coping mechanism. Emotions like stress, anxiety, loneliness, boredom, sadness, or frustration may lead individuals to turn to pornography for temporary relief or distraction.

Thought Triggers: These are particular thoughts or mental associations that evoke the urge to engage in the addictive behavior. For example, fantasizing about explicit content or reminiscing about past experiences with pornography can be thought triggers.

2. Recognizing Triggers:

To identify triggers effectively, individuals need to engage in self-awareness and introspection. Keeping a journal or recording thoughts and emotions before and after consuming pornography can help identify patterns and common triggers. Paying attention to situations and emotions that precede the urge can provide valuable insights.

3. Developing Coping Strategies:

Once triggers are identified, individuals can develop coping strategies to manage them effectively. The goal is to replace the harmful behavior with healthier alternatives. Here are some strategies to consider:

- Avoidance: If certain situations or environments trigger the urge to consume pornography, avoid those triggers whenever possible. For example, limit time spent in private spaces where pornography was previously accessed.
- Substitution: Replace the addictive behavior with healthier alternatives. Engage in activities that provide pleasure, relaxation, or a sense of accomplishment, such as exercise, reading, or spending time with loved ones.
- Mindfulness: Practice mindfulness techniques to become aware of triggering thoughts or emotions

without acting on them. Mindfulness allows individuals to observe their urges without judgment and choose healthier responses.

- Reach Out for Support: When experiencing emotional triggers, seek support from friends, family, or support groups. Talking about your emotions can provide relief and help you process difficult feelings.
- Develop Coping Rituals: Create rituals that help you cope with triggers. This could be a brief meditation or deep breathing exercise when you encounter triggering situations or emotions.

4. Addressing Underlying Issues:

Identifying triggers can also reveal underlying emotional or psychological issues that contribute to the addiction. Addressing these underlying issues through therapy or counseling can be an essential part of the recovery process.

By recognizing and addressing triggers, individuals can take proactive steps to manage their responses and reduce the hold that pornography addiction has on their lives. Over time, with self-awareness and consistent practice of healthy coping strategies, individuals can break free from pornography's grip and build a more fulfilling and balanced life.

6. Develop Healthy Coping Mechanisms: Find healthy alternatives to cope with stress, negative emotions, or boredom. Engage in activities such as exercise, meditation, hobbies, or spending quality time with loved ones to replace the habit of consuming pornography.Pornography addiction often becomes a coping mechanism to deal with stress, negative emotions, boredom, or other life challenges. Breaking free from this addiction requires finding healthier ways to cope with these triggers and emotions. Developing healthy coping mechanisms is essential for managing cravings and redirecting your focus towards more constructive and fulfilling activities.

Examples of Healthy Coping Mechanisms:

1. Exercise: Physical activity, such as jogging, cycling, or yoga, can release endorphins, which are natural mood boosters. Regular exercise can reduce stress and provide a healthier outlet for managing emotions.
2. Meditation and Mindfulness: Practicing meditation or mindfulness techniques can help you become more aware of your thoughts and

emotions without judgment. Mindfulness can reduce anxiety and help you manage cravings more effectively.

3. Engaging in Hobbies: Pursue hobbies and activities that you enjoy and that bring you a sense of accomplishment. Whether it's painting, writing, playing an instrument, or gardening, hobbies can be a positive way to invest your time and energy.

4. Socializing and Support: Spend time with friends, family, or supportive individuals who understand your struggles and offer encouragement. Socializing can provide a sense of belonging and alleviate feelings of loneliness or isolation.

5. Creative Expression: Engage in creative outlets like writing in a journal, drawing, or expressing your emotions through art. Creative expression can be therapeutic and help process complex emotions.

6. Mindful Technology Use: Be conscious of your technology use and seek entertainment or educational content that aligns with your values and interests rather than engaging in pornography.

7. Reading and Learning: Dive into books, articles, or educational content on subjects that interest

you. Continuous learning can be fulfilling and provide a sense of growth and accomplishment.

8. Volunteering: Helping others and contributing to your community can be gratifying. Volunteering allows you to shift the focus away from yourself and toward making a positive impact on others.

9. Seeking Professional Help: If managing your triggers and emotions proves challenging, consider seeking support from a therapist or counselor. They can help you explore underlying issues and provide guidance in developing effective coping strategies.

Experiment and Find What Works for You:

It's important to experiment with different coping mechanisms and find what works best for you. What works for one person may not necessarily work for another. Be patient with yourself as you explore different approaches, and don't be discouraged if some techniques take time to become effective.

Mindset Shift:

Breaking free from pornography addiction involves a mindset shift, recognizing that there are healthier and more constructive ways to cope with life's challenges. Embrace the journey of discovering positive coping mechanisms, and celebrate each step you take towards a healthier and more fulfilling life. Over time, with consistent effort and support, these healthy coping mechanisms can become a natural and empowering part of your daily life.

7. Limit Access to Pornography: Take practical steps to limit access to explicit content. Use website blockers, parental controls, or other tools that restrict your access to adult content.Limiting access to pornography is a practical and effective strategy to reduce temptation and break the cycle of addiction. When individuals struggling with pornography addiction create barriers to accessing explicit content, it becomes easier to resist the urge to engage in the habit. Here are some ways to limit access to pornography:

1. Website Blockers: Use website blocking software or browser extensions that prevent access to adult websites. Many such tools are available, and they allow individuals to set custom filters to block explicit content.

2. Parental Controls: If the issue is with a young adult or teenager, parents can set up parental controls on devices to block access to inappropriate content.

3. Accountability Software: Install accountability software that tracks internet usage and sends reports to a trusted friend, family member, or support group. Knowing that someone is monitoring their online activities can provide an added incentive to stay away from explicit content.

4. Change Browsing Habits: Be mindful of the times and situations when you are most likely to seek out pornography. Avoid using devices in private or during vulnerable moments.

5. Modify Social Media Use: Some social media platforms might expose users to explicit content inadvertently. Consider unfollowing accounts or pages that frequently share or promote adult material.

6. Limit Device Usage: Reduce the amount of time spent on devices that have access to explicit content. This can be particularly helpful during vulnerable periods, such as late at night.

7. Create a Porn-Free Environment: Remove explicit material from your devices, delete saved content, and avoid storing explicit files or links.

The Importance of Limiting Access:

Limiting access to pornography is crucial because it disrupts the automatic response to seek out explicit content when facing triggers or cravings. By creating physical and digital barriers, individuals have a moment to pause and reconsider their actions, making it easier to choose healthier alternatives. This strategy is particularly effective in the early stages of recovery when cravings may be strong and self-control might be challenging.

Complementing with Other Strategies:

Limiting access to pornography works best when combined with other strategies, such as developing healthy coping mechanisms, seeking support, and setting clear goals. Breaking free from pornography addiction often requires a multi-faceted approach that addresses the emotional, psychological, and behavioral aspects of the addiction.

Remember that limiting access to pornography is not a one-time action but an ongoing effort. Staying committed to implementing these strategies and seeking support can significantly increase the chances of successful recovery and pave the way to a healthier and more fulfilling life.

8. Create Structure and Routine: Establishing a daily routine can help you stay focused and avoid idle

moments that might trigger the temptation to consume pornography.Establishing a structured daily routine can be a powerful tool in breaking free from pornography addiction. A structured schedule helps create a sense of order and purpose, reducing idle moments that might trigger the temptation to consume explicit content. Here's why creating structure and routine is beneficial:

1. Occupying Time and Mind: A structured routine fills your day with planned activities and tasks. When your time and mind are occupied with meaningful activities, there is less room for thoughts or urges related to pornography consumption.

2. Reducing Triggers: A routine can help you identify and reduce triggers that lead to porn consumption. By planning your day, you can avoid or minimize situations or emotions that might prompt the desire to engage in the addictive behavior.

3. Forming New Habits: Replacing the habit of watching pornography with healthier activities requires forming new habits. A structured routine allows you to establish positive habits, such as exercising, pursuing hobbies, or spending quality time with loved ones.

4. Enhancing Self-Discipline: Following a routine requires self-discipline and commitment. By adhering to

your daily schedule, you develop a sense of control and discipline, which can be empowering in overcoming addiction.

5. Building Momentum: A structured routine creates a sense of momentum and accomplishment. Each time you complete a planned activity, you gain a sense of achievement, reinforcing your motivation to continue on the path to recovery.

6. Reducing Boredom: Boredom can be a trigger for addictive behaviors. A well-structured routine provides a variety of activities, reducing the likelihood of falling into the trap of pornography consumption out of boredom.

Tips for Creating a Structured Routine:

1. Plan Ahead: Plan your day in advance, allocating time for work, study, self-care, hobbies, exercise, and other activities that bring you joy and fulfillment.
2. Set Realistic Goals: Ensure your routine is achievable and realistic. Setting unrealistic expectations can lead to frustration and discouragement.
3. Include Accountability: Share your routine with a friend, family member, or support group.

Accountability can help you stay committed to following the schedule.

4. Be Flexible: While structure is essential, be open to adjustments when necessary. Life can be unpredictable, and flexibility allows you to adapt your routine to unexpected events.

5. Celebrate Achievements: Acknowledge and celebrate your accomplishments throughout the day. Celebrating progress reinforces positive behavior and motivates you to continue on your journey.

6. Practice Self-Compassion: Be kind to yourself if you deviate from the routine occasionally. It's normal to have setbacks, and self-compassion helps you stay focused on moving forward.

Creating a structured routine is not about filling every minute of your day but rather about providing a framework to guide your actions and choices. It helps you regain control over your time and energy, allowing you to direct your focus toward healthier activities and breaking free from pornography's grip.

9. Practice Mindfulness: Mindfulness techniques can help you become aware of your thoughts and emotions without judgment. Mindfulness can aid in managing cravings and redirecting your focus to healthier

activities.Mindfulness is a mental practice that involves being fully present and aware of the present moment without judgment. It focuses on observing thoughts, emotions, and physical sensations with curiosity and acceptance. When applied to overcoming pornography addiction, mindfulness can be a powerful tool to manage cravings, cope with triggers, and redirect attention towards healthier behaviors.

How Mindfulness Helps in Overcoming Pornography Addiction:

1. Increased Awareness: Mindfulness allows individuals to become more aware of their thoughts and emotions. By recognizing patterns of triggers and cravings, individuals can interrupt the automatic response of seeking pornography and choose healthier alternatives.
2. Non-Judgmental Observation: Mindfulness encourages observing thoughts and feelings without judgment or self-criticism. This approach helps reduce feelings of shame or guilt associated with the addiction, allowing individuals to approach their recovery with self-compassion.
3. Dealing with Cravings: When cravings arise, mindfulness can help individuals acknowledge the sensations and thoughts without acting on

them impulsively. By observing cravings non-judgmentally, individuals can choose not to engage in the addictive behavior.

4. Emotional Regulation: Mindfulness practices can enhance emotional regulation skills. Instead of using pornography as an escape from emotions, individuals can learn to accept and manage their emotions effectively through mindfulness techniques.

5. Refocusing Attention: By training the mind to stay present, mindfulness can help redirect attention from urges to consume pornography towards more positive and productive activities.

Practicing Mindfulness:

Mindfulness can be practiced in various ways, including:

- Meditation: Engaging in formal meditation practices, such as focused breathing or body scans, to develop mindfulness skills.
- Mindful Breathing: Paying attention to the breath, noticing the sensation of inhaling and exhaling, and bringing attention back to the breath when the mind wanders.

- Mindful Awareness: Being fully present in everyday activities, such as eating, walking, or listening, without letting the mind wander.
- Mindfulness Apps and Resources: Utilizing mindfulness apps or guided meditation recordings that provide structured practices to support your journey.

Incorporating Mindfulness into Recovery:

Mindfulness is a skill that takes practice, patience, and consistency. Integrating mindfulness into your daily routine can be beneficial in overcoming pornography addiction. Consider the following steps:

1. Start Small: Begin with short mindfulness sessions and gradually increase the duration as you become more comfortable.
2. Be Consistent: Set aside time each day for mindfulness practice, even if it's just a few minutes.
3. Practice Non-Judgment: During mindfulness, let go of judgment towards yourself or your thoughts. Accept thoughts and emotions as they are without attaching value or criticism.

4. Stay Patient: Developing mindfulness skills takes time, so be patient with yourself as you learn and grow.

Incorporating mindfulness into your recovery journey can enhance self-awareness, self-compassion, and emotional regulation, making it a valuable tool in overcoming pornography addiction and promoting overall well-being.

10. Seek Professional Help: If the addiction is severe or difficult to manage on your own, consider seeking help from a therapist or counselor specializing in sexual addiction. Professional support can offer tailored strategies and guidance.When dealing with pornography addiction, seeking professional help from a therapist, counselor, or support group that specializes in sexual addiction can be immensely beneficial. Here's why professional help is an essential strategy in overcoming addiction:

1. Specialized Expertise: Professionals with experience in sexual addiction understand the complexities of addiction, including the role of pornography in the lives of individuals. They can provide tailored strategies and interventions based on your unique circumstances.

2. Non-Judgmental Environment: Therapy and counseling provide a safe and non-judgmental space for individuals to discuss their struggles with pornography addiction openly. This allows you to explore underlying issues and emotions that may be contributing to the addiction.

3. Identifying Triggers and Coping Mechanisms: A professional can help you identify the triggers that lead to pornography consumption and develop healthier coping mechanisms to manage stress and negative emotions.

4. Accountability and Support: Having a therapist or counselor as an accountability partner can help you stay focused on your goals and track your progress. They can provide support and encouragement throughout your recovery journey.

5. Addressing Underlying Issues: Often, pornography addiction is a symptom of underlying emotional, psychological, or relational issues. A professional can help you address these root causes, which is crucial for sustainable recovery.

6. Relapse Prevention: Professionals can assist in developing relapse prevention strategies to manage cravings and avoid returning to old habits. They can

equip you with tools to navigate challenging situations and maintain progress.

7. Group Support: Support groups for sexual addiction can provide a sense of belonging and understanding. Connecting with others who have experienced similar struggles can reduce feelings of isolation and provide valuable insights.

8. Building Resilience: Through therapy or counseling, you can learn resilience skills to cope with setbacks, strengthen your determination, and develop healthier coping mechanisms.

9. Tailored Treatment Plans: Every individual's addiction journey is unique. Professionals can create personalized treatment plans that consider your specific needs, strengths, and challenges.

10. Long-Term Recovery: Seeking professional help increases the likelihood of long-term recovery from pornography addiction. Professional support can help you build the skills and mindset necessary to maintain a healthy, porn-free life.

It's important to remember that seeking professional help is not a sign of weakness but a courageous step toward healing and growth. Professionals are trained to support individuals in their recovery and offer guidance without judgment. Whether you choose individual therapy, group counseling, or a combination of both, the support and guidance of a professional can significantly enhance your journey to breaking free from pornography's grip and regaining control of your life.

11. Celebrate Progress: Recognize and celebrate the progress you make along the way. Breaking free from pornography's grip is a challenging process, and acknowledging your achievements can boost your motivation.Overcoming pornography addiction is a significant and challenging undertaking, and it's essential to acknowledge and celebrate the progress made along the journey. Celebrating progress serves as a form of positive reinforcement, motivating individuals to continue their efforts and stay committed to their recovery goals. Here are some reasons why celebrating progress is crucial:

1. Boosts Motivation: Recognizing and celebrating the steps taken towards recovery can boost motivation and self-confidence. When individuals see their efforts yielding positive results, they are more likely to stay committed to their goals.

2. Builds Self-Efficacy: Self-efficacy refers to an individual's belief in their ability to achieve their goals.

Celebrating progress reinforces the belief that overcoming addiction is possible, empowering individuals to take on new challenges with confidence.

3. Counteracts Negativity: Breaking free from addiction is not a linear process, and setbacks may occur. Celebrating progress helps counteract negative emotions and self-criticism that may arise after setbacks, providing a more balanced perspective on the journey.

4. Provides Perspective: Addiction recovery can be a long and arduous process, and individuals may feel overwhelmed by the distance still to be covered. Celebrating progress allows them to appreciate how far they've come and stay focused on the positive steps taken.

5. Creates Positive Reinforcement: Celebrating progress creates positive reinforcement for the desired behavior. When individuals see that their efforts are rewarded and acknowledged, they are more likely to continue engaging in healthy behaviors and maintaining their commitment to recovery.

6. Acknowledges Hard Work: Overcoming addiction requires dedication, effort, and perseverance. Celebrating progress acknowledges the hard work individuals put into their recovery journey, validating their efforts and commitment.

How to Celebrate Progress:

Celebrating progress doesn't have to be extravagant; simple gestures and acknowledgments can be meaningful and effective. Here are some ways to celebrate progress while breaking free from pornography addiction:

1. Self-Acknowledgment: Take a moment to recognize your efforts and achievements. You can journal about your progress or simply give yourself positive affirmations.
2. Set Milestones: Break down your recovery journey into smaller milestones and celebrate each achievement. It could be completing a certain number of days without pornography or achieving a personal goal related to recovery.
3. Reward Yourself: Treat yourself to something you enjoy whenever you reach a milestone. It could be spending time doing a favorite activity, buying something special, or pampering yourself with self-care.
4. Share Your Progress: Share your successes with a supportive friend, family member, or support group. Their encouragement and acknowledgment can be highly motivating.

5. Visual Reminders: Create visual reminders of your progress, such as a progress chart or a vision board, to reinforce your commitment and achievements.

Remember that celebrating progress is not about perfection but rather about acknowledging the effort and determination put forth in the journey of recovery. By celebrating the steps taken and staying positive, individuals can build momentum, maintain resilience, and continue moving forward toward a healthier and fulfilling life.

12. Be Kind to Yourself: Overcoming addiction takes time and effort. Be patient and compassionate with yourself during this process, and don't be too hard on yourself if you experience setbacks.Breaking free from pornography addiction can be a challenging and emotional journey. It's essential to practice self-compassion and kindness throughout the process. Here's why being kind to yourself is crucial:

1. Non-Judgmental Attitude: Addiction recovery is not a linear path, and setbacks are a normal part of the process. Instead of being self-critical or judgmental when facing challenges, adopt a non-judgmental attitude. Understand that addiction is complex, and progress may take time.

2. Avoiding Shame and Guilt: Shame and guilt are common emotions experienced by individuals struggling with addiction. However, dwelling on these negative feelings can hinder progress and perpetuate the cycle of addiction. Being kind to yourself involves acknowledging that you are human and that everyone faces struggles.

3. Motivation and Resilience: Practicing self-compassion fosters a positive mindset, which can increase motivation and resilience during the recovery journey. When you treat yourself with kindness, you are more likely to stay committed to your goals and overcome challenges.

4. Embracing Imperfections: Nobody is perfect, and it's essential to recognize that setbacks and mistakes are natural parts of the recovery process. Embracing your imperfections and treating yourself with understanding can help you bounce back from setbacks and continue on the path to recovery.

5. Positive Reinforcement: Celebrating even the smallest victories along the way can reinforce positive behaviors and progress. Acknowledging your efforts and achievements can boost your self-esteem and make you more determined to stay on track.

6. Cultivating Self-Love: Breaking free from addiction involves reshaping your relationship with yourself.

Practicing self-compassion and kindness is a way to cultivate self-love and acceptance. Building a positive self-image can be a powerful foundation for lasting change.

7. Encouraging Growth: Addiction recovery is not just about abstaining from harmful behaviors but also about personal growth and transformation. Being kind to yourself means recognizing your capacity for change and embracing the journey of self-improvement.

8. Reducing Stress: Addiction recovery can be stressful, and self-compassion can help reduce stress levels. When you are kind to yourself, you are less likely to internalize stress and more likely to adopt healthier coping mechanisms.

9. Seeking Help and Support: Being kind to yourself means recognizing when you need help and being open to seeking support from others. Whether it's professional counseling, support groups, or leaning on loved ones, reaching out for assistance is a sign of self-compassion.

10. Maintaining Perspective: Being kind to yourself involves maintaining perspective and avoiding self-criticism. You are not defined by your addiction, and your journey to recovery is a testament to your strength and resilience.

Remember that addiction recovery is a challenging process, but treating yourself with kindness and compassion can make it more manageable and rewarding. Embrace the idea that you deserve support, understanding, and love, and use that foundation to create a healthier and more fulfilling life free from pornography addiction.

Remember that breaking free from pornography addiction is a personal journey, and everyone's experience is unique. Be persistent, stay committed to your goals, and celebrate each step forward on the path to recovery. With determination, support, and the right strategies, it is possible to reclaim control of your life and create a healthier and more fulfilling future.

Chapter 5

Building a Supportive Community

Creating Safe Spaces for Healing and Growth

Creating safe spaces for healing and growth is essential for individuals seeking to overcome challenges, traumas, or addictions. These spaces provide an environment where individuals can feel supported, understood, and empowered to work towards personal growth and well-being. Here are some key elements and strategies for establishing safe spaces:

1. Non-Judgmental and Empathetic Environment:

A safe space should be free from judgment and criticism. People should feel comfortable expressing their thoughts, feelings, and experiences without fear of being judged or misunderstood. Practicing empathy, actively listening, and validating others' emotions are crucial in creating such an environment.

2. Confidentiality and Trust:

Confidentiality is vital in establishing a safe space. Individuals need to trust that what they share within the space will be kept confidential and not used against them. This trust encourages openness and honesty, essential for healing and growth.

3. Respect for Diversity:

A safe space should be inclusive and respectful of diverse backgrounds, experiences, and perspectives. Respecting each person's unique journey fosters a sense of belonging and acceptance.

4. Setting Boundaries and Guidelines:

Establish clear boundaries and guidelines for communication and behavior within the space. Boundaries help create a safe structure and prevent harmful or triggering interactions.

5. Supportive Community:

Encourage a sense of community and support among participants. Knowing that others are going through similar struggles or experiences can provide comfort and validation, reducing feelings of isolation.

6. Professional Guidance (When Appropriate):

In certain healing spaces, such as therapy groups, having a trained facilitator or therapist can provide valuable guidance and structure. Professional support ensures that the space remains focused on growth and healing goals.

7. Encouraging Vulnerability and Authenticity:

Promote an atmosphere where vulnerability and authenticity are welcomed and valued. Being open about one's struggles and experiences can foster deeper connections and facilitate healing.

8. Mindfulness and Emotional Safety:

Encourage mindfulness practices and emotional safety. Mindfulness can help individuals stay present and grounded, while emotional safety ensures that participants feel secure in expressing their emotions.

9. Positive Reinforcement and Recognition:

Recognize and celebrate progress and growth. Positive reinforcement reinforces positive behaviors and encourages individuals to continue their healing journey.

10. Flexibility and Adaptability:

Allow for flexibility and adaptability in the space to meet the evolving needs of participants. Different individuals may require different approaches to healing and growth.

11. Commitment to Growth and Learning:

Promote a culture of continuous growth and learning within the space. Encourage participants to learn from each other's experiences and explore new perspectives and strategies for healing.

12. Self-Care and Compassion:

Emphasize the importance of self-care and self-compassion. Healing can be a challenging process, and individuals need to prioritize their well-being throughout the journey.

Creating safe spaces for healing and growth requires ongoing effort and commitment from all participants. When individuals feel supported, respected, and understood, they can explore and address their challenges, traumas, or addictions more effectively, ultimately leading to personal growth, resilience, and positive change.

Supporting Each Other in the Fight Against Porn Addiction

Supporting each other in the fight against porn addiction is crucial for fostering a caring and understanding community. Here are some ways individuals can offer support and encouragement to those who are struggling with porn addiction:

1. Listen Without Judgment:

Be a compassionate and non-judgmental listener when someone opens up about their struggle with porn addiction. Avoid criticism or blame and instead offer understanding and empathy.

2. Educate Yourself:

Take the time to educate yourself about porn addiction, its impact, and the challenges individuals face while trying to overcome it. Knowledge and awareness can help you provide more informed and supportive assistance.

3. Encourage Seeking Help:

Encourage individuals struggling with porn addiction to seek professional help or join support groups specializing in sexual addiction. Therapy and support networks can provide valuable resources and guidance on the journey to recovery.

4. Be Patient and Understanding:

Recovery from addiction takes time and effort. Be patient and understanding, and avoid putting pressure on someone to recover quickly. Acknowledge that it's a challenging process and offer support throughout their journey.

5. Celebrate Progress:

Recognize and celebrate the progress made by individuals in their fight against porn addiction. Acknowledge their efforts, no matter how small, and reinforce positive behaviors and achievements.

6. Offer Accountability:

Be willing to hold individuals accountable for their actions, but do so with kindness and empathy. Accountability can be a powerful motivator for staying on track with recovery goals.

7. Be Available for Support:

Make yourself available for support whenever needed. Let individuals know that you are there to listen, offer encouragement, or accompany them to support group meetings, if they wish.

8. Promote Healthy Coping Mechanisms:

Encourage the development of healthy coping mechanisms and alternatives to dealing with stress and negative emotions. Suggest activities that can divert their attention away from triggers and towards more positive outlets.

9. Create a Judgment-Free Environment:

Foster a judgment-free environment where individuals feel safe and supported. This creates a space for open communication and vulnerability, which are essential in the recovery process.

10. Practice Self-Care:

Supporters also need to take care of their own well-being. Caring for yourself allows you to be more present and effective in offering support to others.

11. Be Respectful of Boundaries:

Respect the boundaries of individuals in their recovery journey. Some may need space and time to work through their challenges, while others may welcome more active support.

12. Encourage Celebrating Victories:

Celebrate not only major milestones but also everyday victories. Each step towards recovery is significant, and recognizing progress can boost confidence and determination.

By supporting each other in the fight against porn addiction, individuals can foster a sense of community and understanding. Creating an environment of compassion and empathy can make a significant difference in the recovery process, helping individuals overcome challenges and develop healthier relationships with themselves and others.

Conclusion

As you reach the final pages of "Overcoming Porn Addiction for Young Adults: A Guide to Breaking Free and Understanding Yourself," I want to take a moment to commend you on your courage and commitment. The journey you've undertaken is no small feat. Confronting addiction, delving deep into self-understanding, and striving for a better, healthier life requires strength, resilience, and a willingness to face some of the most challenging aspects of your existence. You've demonstrated all of these qualities and more.

Look back at the path you've traveled through this book. From understanding the nature of porn addiction and recognizing its impact on your life to learning practical strategies for breaking free and fostering a deeper connection with yourself, you've covered significant ground. You've taken steps to identify your triggers, developed healthier coping mechanisms, and cultivated a sense of self-compassion that will continue to support you on your journey.

Throughout this book, we've emphasized the importance of understanding – not just of addiction, but of yourself. This understanding is the foundation upon which lasting change is built. By gaining insight into your thoughts, emotions, and behaviors, you've empowered yourself to make conscious choices that align with your true values and aspirations. This newfound awareness is a powerful tool that will serve you well beyond the realm of addiction.

Breaking free from addiction is not a one-time event but an ongoing process. There will be challenges ahead, and there may be moments of doubt or difficulty. But remember, every step you've taken has equipped you with the knowledge, tools, and resilience to face these challenges head-on. Embrace the future with confidence, knowing that you have the strength to navigate whatever comes your way.
One of the key themes we've explored is the importance of connection. Addiction often thrives in isolation, but recovery flourishes in community. Continue to seek out and nurture supportive relationships. Whether it's through support groups, therapy, or trusted friends and family, building a network of understanding and encouragement is crucial for maintaining your progress.

Take time to celebrate your successes, no matter how small they may seem. Each victory, each moment of clarity, and each step towards a healthier life is worth acknowledging. Celebrate the fact that you've chosen to take control of your life and to invest in your well-being. These achievements are testament to your determination and resilience.

As you move forward, remember to treat yourself with kindness and compassion. Recovery is a journey, and it's natural to encounter ups and downs along the way. When setbacks occur, view them as opportunities for growth rather than failures. Treat yourself with the same understanding and patience that you would offer to a close friend.

The tools and strategies you've learned in this book are just the beginning. Continue to explore new ways to support your growth and well-being. Whether it's through mindfulness practices, creative pursuits, physical activities, or new forms of self-expression, find what resonates with you and integrate it into your daily life.

Above all, this book is a message of hope. It's a reminder that no matter how daunting the struggle may seem, recovery is possible. You have the power within you to break free from addiction and to build a life that reflects your true self. You are not defined by your past, but by the choices you make moving forward.

Final Thoughts

Thank you for allowing me to be a part of your journey. Writing this book has been a labor of love, and my greatest hope is that it has provided you with the guidance, support, and inspiration you need to overcome porn addiction and to understand yourself better. Remember, you are not alone. There is a community of individuals who share your journey and who believe in your ability to achieve lasting change.

As you close this book, carry with you the lessons you've learned, the insights you've gained, and the confidence that you have the strength to overcome any challenge. Your journey of breaking free and understanding yourself continues, and the possibilities for your future are boundless.

Here's to your continued growth, healing, and self-discovery. You have the power to create the life you desire, one step at a time.